27729214

STRATEGIC ISSUES IN
Health Care
Management

STRATEGIC ISSUES IN
Health Care
Management

Edited by
M. MALEK
J. RASQUINHA
P. VACANI
University of St Andrews, Fife, Scotland

JOHN WILEY & SONS
Chichester · New York · Brisbane · Toronto · Singapore

Other Wiley Editorial Offices

John Wiley & Sons, Inc., 605 Third Avenue,
New York, NY 10158-0012, USA

Jacaranda Wiley Ltd, G.P.O. Box 859, Brisbane,
Queensland 4001, Australia

John Wiley & Sons (Canada) Ltd, 22 Worcester Road,
Rexdale, Ontario M9W 1L1, Canada

John Wiley & Sons (SEA) Pte Ltd, 37 Jalan Pemimpin #05-04,
Block B, Union Industrial Building, Singapore 2057

British Library Cataloguing in Publication Data

A catalogue record for this book is available from the British Library

ISBN 0 471 93964 1

Produced from camera-ready copy supplied by the Editors
Printed and bound in Great Britain by Bookcraft (Bath) Ltd

ERRATUM

Strategic Issues in Health Care Management

Edited by
M. Malek, J. Rasquinha and P. Vacani

ISBN 0-471-93964-1
©John Wiley & Sons Ltd 1993

Please note that the figures on pages 111 and 249
have been transposed.
We apologise for any inconvenience this may cause.

Contents

SECTION III NATIONAL STANDARD AND
PERFORMANCE EVALUATION

SECTION IV HOSPITAL AND COMMUNITY CARE

List of Contributors

Toni Ashton

School of Medicine,
University of Auckland, New Zealand

Lawton Burns

Department of Management and Policy,
University of Arizona, USA

Ewart Carson

Department of Systems Science,
City University, London

Jon Chilingerian

Heller School for Advanced Studies,
Brandeis University, USA

W.A. Corbett

Gastrointestinal Unit, Department of Surgery,
Middlesborough General Hospital, Cleveland

Derek Cramp

Health Management Group,
Dept. of Systems Science, City University, London

J. Dalhuysen

Faculty of Family Medicine,
Nijmegen University, Limburg, The Netherlands

Martin Den Hartog

Department of Health Economics,
University of Limburg, The Netherlands

Frank Denton

Department of Economics,
McMaster University, Ontario, Canada

Victoria Doyle

Department of Systems Science,
City University, London

Claibourne Dungy   *Department of Paediatrics,*
                            University of Iowa, USA

Chris Evans   *Department of Management,*
                            University of St Andrews

Amiram Gafni   *Centre for Health Economics and Policy Analysis,*
                            Department of Clinical Epidemiology & Biostatistics,
                            McMaster University, Ontario, Canada

Jeanne Goche   *University of Iowa Hospitals and Clinics, USA*

David Grant   *University of Dundee*

Richard Grol   *Faculty of Family Medicine,*
                            Nijmegen University, Limburg, The Netherlands

Meindert Haveman   *Department of Epidemiology,*
                            University of Limburg, The Netherlands

Valerie Iles   *Health Management Group, Dept. of Systems Science,*
                            City University, London

Richard Janssen   *Department of Health Economics,*
                            University of Limburg, The Netherlands

Jurgen John   *GSF-Institut fur Medizinische Informatik und*
                            Systemforschung, Neuherberg, Germany

Mariann Krall   *University of Iowa Hospitals and Clinics, USA*

John Kyriopoulos   *Department of Health Economics,*
                            Athens School of Public Health, Greece

Marion McMurdo   *University of Dundee*

Mo Malek   *Department of Management,*
                            University of St Andrews

Javier Martinez   *Liverpool School of Tropical Medicine, Liverpool*

Andre Meijer   *Faculty of Health Sciences,*
                            Rijksuniversiteit Limburg, The Netherlands

Francois Mennerat

Université Claude Bernard, France

H. Mokkink

Faculty of Family Medicine,
Nijmegen University, Limburg, The Netherlands

Dimitris Niakas

Department of Health Economics,
Athens School of Public Health, Greece

Wim Nuijens

Deptartment of Policy and Research,
Association. of Dutch Sick Funds, The Netherlands

Stanislaw Orzeszyna

Unit of Monitoring, Evaluation & Projection
Methodology,
World Health Organization, Switzerland

Klaus Piwernetz

GSF-Institut fur Medizinische Informatik und
Systemforschung, Neuherberg, Germany

Svein Raknes

Ministry of Health and Social Affairs, Norway

Joe Rasquinha

Department of Management,
University of St Andrews

Zillyham Rojas

Liverpool School of Tropical Medicine, Liverpool

Peter Sandiford

Liverpool School of Tropical Medicine, Liverpool

Stephen Sapirie

Unit of Monitoring, Evaluation & Projection
Methodology,
World Health Organization, Switzerland

Walter Satzinger

GSF-Institut fur Medizinische Informatik und
Systemforschung, Neuherberg, Germany

Jill Schofield

Aston Business School,
Aston University, Birmingham

Veron Schrijnemaekers

University of Limburg, Netherlands

James Seldon

Division of Business, Computing and Mathematics,
University College of the Cariboo, Canada

David Simpson   *School of Computing and Mathematics,*
                             University of Teeside, Cleveland

Derek Simpson   *School of Computing & Mathematics,*
                            University of Teeside, Cleveland

Peter Sonksen   *Dept. of Endocrinology and Chemical Pathology,*
                            St Thomas's Hospital, London

Byron Spencer   *Department of Economics,*
                            McMaster University, Ontario, Canada

Greg Stoddart   *Dept. of Clinical Epidemiology and Biostatistics,*
                            McMaster University, Ontario, Canada

Ala Szczepura   *Warwick Business School,*
                            University of Warwick, Coventry

Florence Taboulet   *Service de Droit et Economie Pharmaceutiques,*
                            France

Michel Thuriaux   *Unit of Strengthening of Epidemiology and Statistical*
                            Services,
                            World Health Organisation, Switzerland

Paul Vacani   *Universities of St Andrews and Dundee, Scotland*

Martien Van Tits   *Institute of Social Research,*
                            Tilburg University, The Netherlands

Douglas Wholey   *Department of Social and Decision Sciences,*
                            Carnegie Mellon University, USA

Antonius Zwaard   *Faculty of Family Medicine,*
                            Nijmegen University, Limburg, The Netherlands

Acknowledgements

Several individuals have contributed directly or indirectly to the development of this volume. We wish to thank Julian Crowe, Elin Kaafjeld and Farzana Malik for their general help in the preparation of the book. Thanks are also due to our colleagues in the Pharmacoeconomics Research Centre in both Dundee and St Andrews Universities, among them special thanks goes to Chris Evans. We should also like to thank Verity Waite and Lucy Jepson of John Wiley & Sons who persevered with us throughout the project.

Finally, Deirdre Crummey deserves special mention for her careful production of the manuscript. Deirdre joined the team rather late, but soon became an indispensable member, and with her patient and efficient contribution we managed to finish the volume on time.

Preface

This book examines issues which have long been of strategic importance to the organisation and delivery of health services in various countries, with different systems of governmental, political regimes and cultural backgrounds. Many of these issues are not new, and they periodically re-emerge in different guises. This can be taken as a testimony to their resilience, and the critical roles they play in the conceptualisation of health care provision. This book represents a collection of works by clinicians, academics, practitioners, system scientists and others who have worked extensively in these problem areas, and value the cross-fertilisation of ideas.

STRUCTURE OF THE BOOK

The twenty three papers presented in this book are organised in four different sections: Funding Health Care Systems; Resource Planning; National Standards and Performance Evaluation; and Hospital and Community Care. The choice of the parts are arbitrary as some papers cover subject areas which span the boundaries of these sections.

In chapter 1, Mennerat and Taboulet deal with an old question: that of the compatibility of medical and budgetary rationale. The context is the French "Seguin Plan". The plan's objective is to make structural change in the health care system less susceptible to financial fluctuation, whilst at the same time seeking a more egalitarian system. The same question, this time in the context of New Zealand, is raised by Toni Ashton in chapter 2. A regime of co-payments and user charges for publicly funded health services was introduced in February 1992. It is too early to examine the consequences of these changes, but she explains the objectives of the new system and speculates on the likely winners and losers. Van Tits and Nuijens examine the Dutch health care system, which is also in a state of transition. The vehicle this time is decentralisation, aiming at strengthening the co-operation between the insurers and the providers. Insurance, with universal coverage and the freedom to choose any health insurer which they deem appropriate, will introduce a budget deficit which will be met by a per capita premium set by the insurer and acting as an incentive for achieving a greater degree of efficiency.

Section 2 relates to Resource Planning. It includes six papers which discuss the theme and approach from different angles — at times these are in conflict with each other. In chapter 4, Malek *et al* commence the debate, arguing the case for some measure of total system efficiency, which takes into account the scarcity of the resources available. The context of their debate is the developing countries, but the case they present for resource planning is essentially context-free, and thus can equally apply to the developed countries or indeed a sub-system within any country. The question of resource planning is also the subject of Denton *et al,* in their interesting paper, which introduces us to SHARP, a micro computer-based System for Health Area Resource Planning. The system, although devised for the province of Ontario in Canada, has potential for application in other areas. Kyriopoulos and Niakas, in chapter 6, outline the transition and the changes in the imperatives of the Greece Health System during the 1980's. They are primarily concerned with the use of high technology medicine and its diffusion rate between the public and private sector, and the effect it has had on the demand for health services. A different aspect of resource planning and utilisation is the subject of chapter 7, taken up by Rojas *et al.* These authors question the value and appropriateness of the training courses designed in developed countries, for health managers of developing countries. The contrasting model is a problem-based learning approach taught in the local language, with on-site training and using real-life examples, taken from the context of the developing countries with direct relevance. This is an innovative and promising approach to training health managers. In chapter 8 Krall *et al* discuss another innovative strategy in a teaching hospital in the United States, seeking to increase the effectiveness of health care delivery and enhance the quality of care in the ambulatory setting. Seldon and Stoddart, in chapter 9, discuss the value (cost) of technological innovation in health care. They argue that it is not easy to distinguish between cost-saving and cost-increasing technological change and that the tactical need for the (partial) evaluation of the new technology has to be balanced against the strategic benefits of technical advances. This paper bridges the gap between sections (2) and (3)., the latter addresses the area of performance evaluation.

Ala Szczepura in chapter 10 reports the results of an EC funded project, spanning eight European Countries, on Health Care Technology assessment. The results raise important questions regarding the type of the technologies to be assessed and the timing of such assessments. As it has placed emphasis on the harmonisation process by the European Community, Szczepura's paper has some immediate policy implications for the effective utilisation of technology in health care.

In chapter 11, Doyle *et al* use an inter-disciplinary customer supplier model for structuring clinical audit and quality control. This paper, together, with that of Simpson *et al* in chapter 12, although both context-specific, have wider applicability beyond the clinical settings within which the studies have been conducted. In chapter 13 Orzeszyna *et al* discuss the use of an issue-information matrix in the rapid evaluation of health services performance in six developing countries between 1988 and 1991. The method appears to be readily accessible, easy to administer and the information gathered provides a useful source for technical and managerial decision making.   Furthermore, the method is easily transferable to other developing countries.   Acceptance and diffusion of standards are also the subject of the paper by Zwaard and Grol in chapter 14.   The question they address is not how to set up national standards but how to encourage doctors to accept these standards, and to apply them in their day-to-day clinical practice.   The next two papers in chapters 15 and 16 deal with the particularly pressing problem of the care of the elderly patients in developed countries.   McMurdo and Grant, in chapter 15, relay their own experience of the assessment of the quality of medicine for the elderly in Scotland. Schrijnemaekers and Haveman's paper reports on a randomised controlled study on the assessment of the effectiveness of a geriatric unit in the Netherlands.   Chapter 17 by Ilse *et al* concludes Section III by discussing the important issue of bridging the gap between clinical realities and that of strategic decision making.   Some of the issues raised are similar with that of Rojas *et al* in chapter 7, albeit in a different context.

The final section of the volume deals with the delivery of care in the hospital setting.   Janssen and Den Hartog, in chapter 18, take up the subject of Dutch health reforms aimed at improving efficiency in the hospital sector, by the introduction of a market like structure into the system.   British readers will be excused for feeling a sense of deja vu.   The issue of efficiency in managing hospitalised *patients* is again raised in chapter 19 by Burns *et al*.   The authors conceptualise physicians as the managers of a "temporary firm", which aims to provide hospital care for patients admitted.   The results of this extensive study, in the USA, provide a fascinating explanation, highlighting factors affecting inter-physician behaviour.   Treating the hospital as a firm is also the recurrent theme for Svein Raknes's paper set in Norway. This paper ideally should be read in conjunction with the previous chapter.   Satzinger and John, in Chapter 21, deal with another aspect of quality assurance in the German hospitals, whilst in chapter 22 Jill Schofield uses a specific example to highlight the experience of contract negotiation simulation between purchaser and providers within the UK internal market, or as she puts it more aptly, within *quasi*-markets. The volume concludes with a paper from the Netherlands presented by A.W.M. Meijer which raises strategic issues in the municipal services for community care.

Thus, after 23 papers we return full circle to ask questions regarding strategic choice, option and implementation.   The papers presented are fine examples of scholarly works, provide much food for thought, and set many research agenda for the future.

Section I

Funding Health Care Systems

1 Budgetary and Medical Rationale in the French Plan for Rationalisation of Health Expenditures ("Séguin plan")

FRANÇOIS MENNERAT[1] & FLORENCE TABOULET[2]

[1]*G.S. Sante, Université Claude Bernard, France*
[2]*Service de Droit et Economie Pharmaceutiques, France*

The numerous recovery plans that had been successively devised between 1975 and 1986 had a slight and temporary influence on the ascending curve of total medical expenses. Since these plans modified the coverage of ordinary insured people alone, a widening gap separated this population from the fully insured. In 1986, the fully insured constituted 6.2% of the overall population, of which half of them were over 60 who were exonerated from the moderating ticket[1], were responsible for 55.5% of pharmaceutical expenses from health insurance funds, *versus* only 50% in 1980. Faced with a noticeable increase in the number of fully covered people, and, the concentration of expenses over a smaller part of the insured, the Minister of Social Affairs and Employment, Philippe Séguin, undertook what he termed "a progressive action of resetting to rights". His main target was the level of funding of the pharmaceutical expenses for the fully insured. The results of his policy were conclusive, since beyond expectation, approximately 9.4 billion Francs have been saved.

In addition to extending measures such as no longer reimbursing several classes of drugs, the Séguin plan, as it has been termed, introduced more innovative reforms. These reforms turned out to be very efficient. They did not target pharmaceutical products *per se*, but the level of coverage of definite categories of insured people:

---

[1]   The "moderating ticket" represents the part that is not covered by health insurance, and is left to the patient's own expense, or to his complementary health insurance if any. It ranges from 20% to 25% or even 35% for health care practitioners or providers, and from 0% to 60% depending on drugs classes. Even though this kind of measure has never proved its efficacy at such low levels (especially when a complementary health insurance exists), it is supposed to restrain the patient from making excessive use of the health care system.

Strategic Issues in Health Care Management. Edited by M. Malek, J. Rasquinha and P. Vacani
© 1993 John Wiley & Sons Ltd

the so-called "26th disease"[2] which disappeared, to be replaced by the "40 at 40",[3] particularly for patients acknowledged as suffering from a long term disease[4]. Thus the new principle of a clear discrimination between reimbursement of an *exonerating disease* and a less serious *intercurrent disease* was introduced, a principle still applied to-day.

These last two measures clearly aimed to harmonise the rights of the exonerated insured with the non-exonerated (common law) ones. Differentiated coverage for small health hazards was concurrently extended to any insured people, strengthening the concept of "comfort medicines" previously initiated in 1977. Definitively, the plan was an attempt to bound the social privileges granted to patients suffering from long term diseases. In a way, the Séguin plan represented a levelling of rights, an abolishment (in part) of privileges, and consequently, a step towards egalitarianism.

But, equality is not necessarily synonymous to equity. It is obvious that health care needs are, by nature, radically unequal. Must equality be given more importance over solidarity?

Using figures from the *Caisse Nationale d'Assurance-Maladie des Travailleurs Salariés (CNAMTS)*, the supplementary pharmaceutical expenses of the insured in 1987 can be determined as follows:

- F 4,075, for the insured who had lost their right to full coverage,
- F 340[5] to F 1,770, for the insured who had kept it in spite of the changes introduced .

Besides, is it possible, as the new dispositions take for granted to determine *ex-ante* the nature and amount of care being directly derived from long term disease? In other words, can therapeutic practice comply with administrative regulations that are responsible for sorting drugs between three groups? Further, in clinical practice, are the differences between patients suffering from long term disease and the common law insured rigorously reflected in the range of drug prescriptions?

Even though the Seguin Plan seemingly follows an indisputable administrative and budgetary logic, the proposed measures look ambitious from both the social and political points of view, since it remains unknown as to whether therapeutics can strictly follow pre-established schemes. But undeniably the many postulates that the

---

2   Prior to the "Séguin plan", a patient was granted a *full* coverage of *any* expenses in at least two situations: if he suffered from a disease quoted on a list of 25 long term diseases, or, and this was dubbed the 26th disease, his uncovered expenses (the so-called "moderating ticket", cf. supra) exceeded a threshold of F 80.

3   This term means that drugs stamped for 40% reimbursement are effectively reimbursed at this level even for the fully insured.

4   The previous list of 25 long term diseases (*ALD*, for *Affections de Longue Durée*) was extended to 30, with an extra category (called the 31st disease) meant for cases of patients suffering from unlisted serious diseases.

5   Only for the sub-population of beneficiaries of a supplementary allowance called the "19th allowance" in the jargon of the French health insurance fund.

plan supposes cannot be validated until experiments are attempted, and results are forthcoming.

In particular, the analysis of such a plan, (also designed as an incisive policy of demand regulation,) provides potential evidence of an existing relationship between the level of refunding and the consumer's behaviour as a purchaser. The *princeps* effect of the "Plan for Rationalisation of Health Expenses" as it had officially been called, is a dramatic drop in the pharmaceutical expenses that were totally exonerated from any "moderating ticket", and therefore totally covered by the sick-funds. However, until 1986, the average annual increase of these expenses had reached 4.5%, though in 1987, and 1988, an average annual drop of 18.5% was observed.

The expenses exonerated from the "moderating ticket" (EMT expenses) were 54.2% for the first term in 1986, as against only 35.7% for the first term in 1988. Actually the corollary of such a decrease, both in absolute and relative value, is conversely an increase of the expenses of the moderating ticket (WMT expenses) within the coverage of sick-funds. But account must be taken of the various rates of reimbursement applied to these expenses, and that the decrease of EMT expenses exceeded the increase of WMT expenses covered by the sick-funds. It means that beyond a simple transfer from public funding towards households budgets[6], the Séguin plan has also had an impact on health care consumption. This is reflected in the fact that the 1987 expenses presented for reimbursement (i.e. corresponding to the real value of the products purchased) are less by 4% to those forecast by the extrapolation of the trend during the previous years. Therefore, one must disassociate savings linked to the increase of the average moderating ticket, and those linked to the reduction in the increase of medical consumption. *Direct effects* and *induced effects* must then be distinguished. They are estimated at 5.769 billions Francs: nearly half the overall savings achieved and are attributable to a change in the actors' behaviour.

- Physicians being more sensitive to the economic dimension of their activity. It must be remembered that the sick-funds had campaigned for a better use of health care by both the physicians and the patients.
- Patients moderating their demand of care. For some of them the increase in charges has had a dissuasive effect, or in other words, price-elasticity of drugs is relevant.
- The absence of any epidemic of influenza in 1987 and 1988 (as revealed by the usual indicators: number of home visits, consumption of anti-infectious and of respiratory tract drugs, surveys by the GROG, i.e. a network of GPs for the observation of influenza, etc.).

If these savings induced by the absence of winter seasonal pathology can be extrapolated from the data of the previous years , it would seem to be difficult to

---

6   The overall coverage rate was 77% in 1986; it was no more than 71% for the first months
     of 1987, and 68.8% for the first term of 1988.

assess the respective weights of the two above elements. In fact, there appears to be an effect on supply, which is mutually connected with the effect on demand.

Analyses of chronological series of consumption of several therapeutic classes, both in monetary value and in quantities, have been achieved. The data below in table 1, displayed in quantities expressed in number of boxes is extracted from sales statistics by IMS [7].

Table 1. Changes in the overall pharmaceutical market
Cumulative number of boxes sold [8]

	January-August 85	January-August 86	January-August 87
General market	+ 6 %	+ 4 %	- 5 %
40 % reimb. range	+ 8 %	+ 3 %	- 8 %
70 % reimb. range	+ 6 %	+ 8 %	- 0 %

Consumption trends were abruptly reversed in 1987. It is observed that families with a low 40% coverage indicate the greatest fall. In the use of the various therapeutic groups, the dynamics appear very dissimilar and the evidence of phenomenons of substitutions between pharmaceutical specialities have been found.

In order to provide an answer to the cyclical financial imbalance of Social Security, as had been the rationale for previous plans, the Séguin plan was conspicuous, from the nature of several of the reforms it introduced. Some of them could actually be termed structural reforms, in the sense that they entailed changes in the relationships among various actors in the pharmaceutical market, as well as changes in the behaviour of these actors.

The intentions of physicians, pharmacists, medical-advisers[9] and mutual insurance companies have been described, and the impact of adapting to these various actors have been analysed. Hereafter, we will only recall a few developments.

The discrimination between prescriptions relating to exonerating and to intercurrent conditions relies on information interchanges between actors, which implies a *de facto* build up of an information system. Hastily designed, this information system indicates numerous negative attributes, giving way to irrelevant interpretation. It is based, at the patient's request, on a declaration by a physician of his choice. The declaration uses a special form called "Protocole Inter-Régimes

---

7 Informations Médicales et Statistiques, a private company specialised in market studies in the field of health care.

8 Source: Claudine Sapède, "Le plan Séguin: incidences sur la consommation du médicament", Thesis for the Doctorate in Pharmacy, University of Clermont-Ferrand I, December 1987.

9 This profession is very specific to the French health insurance system. Medical advisers are physicians who are appointed by a sick fund, with the function to schematically provide medical advice whenever the funding or reimbursement of care is subject to an assessment of the patient's status in order to discriminate between various levels of rights.

d'Examen Spécial" (PIRES), and is meant to describe the long term exonerating diseases and to establish the framework of a therapeutic programme. It forms the basis of an agreement with the sick-fund through the medium of their medical-adviser. The patient is later provided with a special book of prescription sheets reserved for the treatment of exonerating conditions.

Difficulties originate in the fact that if PIRES is to be considered as a contractual document, only contracting parties are bound, particularly as the patient is concerned, the physician who has written it out alone. On the one hand it can be observed that the physician signatory of the PIRES is himself reluctant to use, as he should do, his ordinary book of prescription sheets. This is because the prescriptions are meant for the treatment of non exonerating conditions, and it is very likely that this behaviour is driven by the pressure of the client-patient. On the other hand, in case of an inpatient stay or in the consultation of a medical specialist, account is seldom taken of the initial contract, since on these occasions each non-contracting partner can pretend with a certain degree of plausibility that he totally ignores its content.

Generally speaking, many prescriptions related to intercurrent conditions are abusively or fraudulently written on a prescription sheet reserved for exonerating conditions. Besides, hospital charges are directly invoiced without a moderating ticket and without questioning the medical-adviser by the form specially devised for this purpose. Thus, the different actors can argue they are sincere and put forward their ignorance of the conditions that have precisely given way to full coverage.

This is facilitated by the absence of regulations allowing for the management of any contentious matters arising from the deviant use of the dispositions meant for long term diseases. The actors' obligations are not clearly stipulated by the law. The functioning of the whole process relies only on rules of good conduct that have been drawn up by the signatories of the national agreement between the sick funds and the physicians, without any coercive measure being contemplated. If, as always, potential for dispute arises about the medical scope of full coverage, the only possible recourse is through professional jurisdiction, which is actually a section of the Medical Council ("Section des Assurances Sociales de l'Ordre des Médecins"), but on the condition that clear evidence exists of abnormal behaviour, and, that the stated excesses were systematic and permanent.

If, on the long term, the Séguin plan seems to have only delayed the continuing increase of health care expenses, it can be imputed, at least in part, to the modalities of its implementation. However, the specificities of the Séguin plan have to be stressed. We have seen that it aimed at slowing down supply through the medium of an action on the demand. Furthermore, this plan has been built on new notions that are capable of unsettling the principles on which health insurance is based in France. In particular, substituting the protection of the person by protecting against illness, and that too a well delineated disease, reveals a swing of the French social protective system from one of solidarity towards one of insurance, with its own logic of differentiating the management of hazards.

2 Charging for Health Services — Some Anecdotes from the Antipodes

TONI ASHTON

University of Auckland, New Zealand

INTRODUCTION

In February 1992, a new regime of user charges for publicly funded health services was introduced into New Zealand, along with proposals for major reform of the public health system (Upton, 1991). The new charging regime included the introduction of charges for hospital services as well as a revamping of existing charges for general practitioner (GP) consultations and pharmaceuticals. The thrust of the changes was to increase charges for higher income groups and to direct these additional funds towards increasing primary care subsidies for those on lower incomes.

The official title of the new system is the "Interim Targeting Regime". This does not imply that user charges will be temporary, indeed the government has made clear its commitment to user charges as an acceptable and appropriate mechanism for funding health services. Rather, the charges are an interim measure until a new system has been developed for setting limits on a family's total annual expenditure on public health services. In the meantime, the intention is to fine tune the charging regime over time and some minor changes have already been made towards this end. After outlining details of the new regime, this paper examines the objectives of the changes and discusses the extent to which these objectives are likely to be met.

THE INTERIM TARGETING REGIME

Charging for primary health services is not a new concept in New Zealand. Since 1941 when subsidies for GP services were first introduced, general practitioners have retained the right to charge whatever additional fee they see fit over and above the fixed subsidy paid by the government. Initially, the subsidy accounted for about 75% of the total price of a consultation but, because the subsidy level has been increased only rarely, its real value became seriously eroded. By 1990, the adult subsidy of $4

Strategic Issues in Health Care Management. Edited by M. Malek, J. Rasquinha and P. Vacani
© 1993 John Wiley & Sons Ltd

accounted for only about 10-15% of the total price of a consultation. On 1 February 1991 the subsidy was abolished completely for everyone except children, the elderly, beneficiaries and those with chronic illnesses (Table 1). The full fee paid by unsubsidised patients now generally falls within the range of NZ$30 - $40[1].

Part-charges for pharmaceuticals were first introduced in 1989. Unlike GP subsidies, the government sets the level of charges rather than the level of the subsidy so that patients pay the same charges throughout the country. These charges were initially very modest (NZ$5 for adults and $2 for the special groups listed above) but were soon increased to $15 and $5 respectively on 1 February 1991 (Table 1).

Details of the new charging regime were announced in the budget on 1 July 1991 (Shipley,1991). Under the new regime, different levels of charges apply for three different income groups, the thresholds for which vary according to family size. Details of the charges which apply to adults (including the elderly) in each income group are given in Table 2. Lower charges apply for children and high users. Maximum annual limits of 15 prescription items, 10 in-patient nights and 5 out-patient visits were placed on the amount of services a family must pay for within in a year. No limit applies to general practitioner consultations although individuals visiting a GP more than 6 times in 6 months for the same medical condition are classified as 'high users' and so are entitled to higher subsidies.

Entitlement to higher subsidies is secured through a new card called the Community Services Card (CSC) which is issued to families in the two lower income groups (Groups 1 and 2). Anyone without a CSC (or a High User Card) is assumed to be in the highest income group (Group 3) and is charged at the highest rate.

The changes had different impacts on different groups of people. The main winners were working adults on very low incomes (Group 1). For this group, charges for GP services and pharmaceuticals fell by $15 and $10 respectively. Beneficiaries were also marginally better off. Adults in Group 2 faced lower charges for primary care but were required to pay new charges for hospital services. For those in Group 3, especially children, all charges increased except for GP services for which they were already being charged the full amount.

The changes were part of more widespread economic and social reforms which were being introduced into New Zealand. These reforms reflected the more-market ideology of governments in recent years, including a general belief in the superiority of self-reliance over community responsibility. But the application of these economic policies to health care was not supported by many in the health sector[2]. The changes in users charges were therefore followed by ardent debate. The introduction of hospital charges was especially contentious, with "free" hospital care having long been viewed as the right of all New Zealanders. Preferences were expressed for an increase in taxes rather than the payment for services through user charges. Some

---

[1]NZ$1.00 = 33p

[2]For example, one group of 31 health professionals and commentators published a critique of the reforms stating that: "Market theory has only limited application to the complex problems of distributing health care and developing community well-being." (Wellington Health Action Committee, p7)

Table 1. GP Subsidies and Pharmaceutical Charges, 1991- 1993

Category of patient	Before 1.2.91 $	1.2.91 to 1.2.92 $	From 1.2.92 Group 1[1] $	Group 2[2] $	Group 3[3] $
		General practitioner subsidy			
Children 0-4	29	25	25	25	15
Children 5+	24	20	20	20	15
Adults	4	0	15	12	0
Beneficiaries	12	12	15	n/a	n/a
Elderly	17	12	15	12	0
High users					
Child 0-4	29	25	25	25	25
Child 5+	24	20	20	20	20
Adult	17	17	17	17	17
		Prescription charges[4]			
			from 1.2.93	from 1.2.93	from 1.2.93
Children 0-4	2	5	5 (3)	5 (3)	20 (15)
Children 5+	2	5	5 (3)	5 (3)	20 (15)
Adults	5	15	5 (3)	7.5 (4)	20 (15)
Beneficiaries	2	5	5 (3)	n/a	n/a
Elderly	2	5	5 (3)	7.5 (4)	20 (15)
High users	2	5	5 (3)	5 (3)	5 (3)

1. Group 1 = Beneficiaries, recipients of student allowances, very low income working adults, and
   families receiving unabated income support.
2. Group 2 = Families receiving partial income support.
3. Group 3 = All others
4. These are maximum charges. Any prescription items costing less than the maximum charge is
   charged at its normal retail price.
n/a: Not applicable as all beneficiaries are in Group 1.

groups encouraged people to express their opposition by refusing to pay the new charges for hospital services.

Perhaps as a result of this debate, some minor changes were made to the proposed charges before they were even introduced. These included the overturning of a proposal to introduce a $2 charge for laboratory tests, and an increase in the GP subsidy for children in Group 3 from zero to $15. Nevertheless, most of the new regime was introduced as originally planned. Subsequent concern about access to primary care encouraged the government to revise the pharmaceutical charges downwards from 1 February 1993 as shown in Table 1. At the same time, the maximum number of charges for prescription items was increased from 15 to 20 per annum per family.

Table 2. Adult subsidies and charges under the new regime

Service	Group1 $	Group 2 $	Group 3 $
GP Consultations[1]	15	12	0
Pharmaceuticals[2]	5	7.50	20
Out-patient[3]	0	19	31
In-patient[3]	0	35	50

1. This is the subsidy level (rather than the charge): additional fee paid by patient is set by each GP.
2. These charges for pharmaceuticals were reduced from 1 February 1993 to $3.00, $4.00 and $15 respectively. At the same time, the maximum limit was raised to 20 prescription items per family per year.
3. Some hospital services are exempt from these charges, including maternity services, mental health services, sexually transmissible disease services, and accident-related services. Those classified as high users do not pay any hospital charges, regardless of their income group.

OBJECTIVES OF THE CHARGES

There appear to be four main objectives of the new regime:

i.   to target resources towards low income groups,
ii.   to reduce cost-shifting from general practice to hospitals,
iii. to achieve greater efficiency in resource use, and
iv.   to reduce government expenditure.

Targeting resources towards low income groups

Prior to the changes, fees for GP services had become increasingly prohibitive for lower income groups, especially working adults who were not entitled to any government subsidy. A major objective behind the rationalisation of charges was therefore to reduce these barriers to access by increasing the subsidisation of both GP services and pharmaceuticals for those in the two lower income groups.

Even with the higher subsidies, the patient charge for a GP consultation for a person in the lowest income group can still be as high as $24 in some areas. Nevertheless, preliminary indications are that utilisation of GP services may have increased slightly for those in Group 1 and fallen for those in Group 3. For social welfare beneficiaries, however, any potential benefits from the small ($3) increase in the general practice subsidy had already been offset by a reduction in the level of social welfare payments just prior to the announcement of the new charging regime.

While the intention was to reduce the financial barriers for low income groups, concerns are now being expressed that problems of access have simply been shifted further up the income scale. The income thresholds for the highest income group (Group 3) are very low (see Figure 1).

For example, a single person living alone and a married couple without children fall into Group 3 if their gross incomes exceed $17,500 and $23,000 respectively. This is well below the average wage which is currently around $30,000. The high level of charges for prescription items for people - especially children - in Group 3 was of particular concern and pharmacists reported a marked increase in the number of patients who failed to uplift prescription items when advised of the charges. This

INCOME ($)

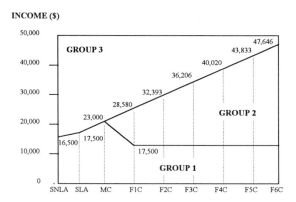

SNLA (Single Not Living Alone), SLA (Single Living Alone), MC (Married Couples),
F1C (Family 1 Child), F2C (Family 2 Children), F3C (Family 3 Children),
F4C (Family 4 Children), F5C (Family 5 Children), F6C (Family 6 Children)

Figure 1. Income thresholds for 3 income groups

will be eased by the downward revision in charges for pharmaceuticals from 1 February 1993 (Table 2). Nevertheless, a bill for an adult attending a general practitioner and being prescribed two prescription items could still be $65 or more.

Whether or not the charging regime will work as intended depends to a large extent on the ability and willingness of families to apply for and use the Community Services Card as intended. Uptake of the card is far from complete, especially for low income people who cannot be traced through the social welfare system and who must therefore apply for the card of their own accord. Problems of uptake and use may stem from lack of information and understanding about the system, from shame or embarrassment at being labelled "poor", or from the fact that many families do not actually know the level of their family income. Even where a family in Group 1 or 2 does have a CSC, some family members may not wish their use of health services to be known by other family members. A further complicating factor is that each family is responsible for keeping track of their total annual service use for the purposes of the maximum annual limits, although individual service providers also keep records.

Use of the family as the unit for determining entitlement is proving difficult to monitor. One (anonymous) administrator reported that the family members included in the CSC is open to "creative interpretation". In some cases, such as where children spend equal time with each of two parents who are separated, there is some confusion about who belongs to which family.

Although family income is the basic unit of assessment, the new charging regime is complicated by the fact that there are two other variables - age and health status - which also determine entitlement. This means that two families in the same income group with equal use of health services may face quite different charges, depending upon the age and health status of the family members who use the service. To illustrate the point, the example given in Table 3 compares two families in Group 3 earning exactly the same income, each with four children of the same age, and each using 12 GP consultations, 12 prescription items, and 12 nights in hospital. In Family 1, each parent visits the GP four times in the year while each of the four children visit only once. In Family 2, two of the children have health problems and so account for all of the family's use of health services. Both of these two children visit the doctor 6 times each within 6 months, have 6 prescription items each (3 at full-rate and 3 after becoming entitled to the subsidy for high users). One of these children also spends 12 nights in hospital. While the annual bill for Family 1 is $992, Family 2 pay only $300. Clearly the objective of ensuring equal access for people on equal incomes has not been reached.

Table 3. Comparison of charges for two families with different patterns of service use

Type of charge	Family 1	Family 2
	$	$
GP Consultations		
Adult	248	nil
Child	64	192
Pharmaceuticals		
Full rate	180	90
High users	nil	18
In-patient	500	nil
Total	$992	$300

This problem of unequal access would be reduced quite significantly if a global stoploss (i.e. a single maximum annual charge per family regardless of the type of service used) could be implemented. Work is currently underway to examine ways of implementing such a system.

In sum, it seems likely that some of the financial barriers to access for low income people have been removed by the new regime. However new problems of access have been introduced, especially for those in the lower income brackets of Group 3.

Reducing cost-shifting

As the real value of GP subsidies has eroded over the years, the incentive has increased for people to use hospital emergency departments for the treatment of minor ailments in preference to a GP who would charge a fee. In an effort to discourage this cost-shifting practice, the charges for out-patient services for Groups 2 and 3 were set at a level that is equal to the national average patient charge for GP services for people in these income groups.

In fact, the inappropriate use of hospital emergency departments had already been significantly reduced prior to the introduction of the new charging regime through improved management practices. Moreover, it is lower income groups (Group 1) who have the greatest financial incentive to seek care from the lowest cost provider and out-patient services remain free for this group. For those in Groups 2 and 3, the incentive to shift cost is only removed as long as GP fees are not much greater than out-patient charges. But many doctors increased their fees soon after the new charges were introduced, in part to compensate for the additional costs associated with administering the new, more complicated, regime. A further difficulty is that the level of GP fees - and hence the incentive to -shift cost- varies quite significantly across the country. In the light of these considerations, it seems unlikely that the inappropriate use of hospitals will be entirely resolved by the new regime.

Achieving greater efficiency in resource use

In explaining the rationale for the new charging regime the government emphasised the need for people to be more aware of the cost of health services, the assumption being that greater efficiency should be achieved if people are discouraged from using services unnecessarily. Almost all empirical studies of user charges support the hypothesis that charges reduce the use of both primary and secondary services (Van de Ven, 1983). However, in New Zealand, about half of the population will be paying the same, or less, for most services under the new regime. Moreover, of the remainder, about half have private health insurance which allows them to claim back part, if not all, of the charge. Therefore any potential efficiency gains through reduced service use are limited to that minority (mostly in Group 3) who face higher charges *and* who do not hold private insurance.

The intention of the government is presumably only to reduce the use of services that are medically unnecessary. However a distinction needs to be made between over-use in the medical sense and over-use in an economic sense. People often do not have the information that require (or are not physically or mentally able) to make an informed decision about the value of services in relation to their particular health needs. A person who is willing and able to pay for a service that is medically unnecessary is still using services efficiently in an economic sense because they value the service at least as much as the price that they have to pay. Similarly a poorer person who is unwilling to pay for a service that is regarded as medically necessary is also using resources efficiently from an economic perspective. Using data from the Rand Health Insurance Experiment in the USA, Lohr et al (1986) reported that utilisation of services that were categorised as highly medically effective declined equally with services categorised as medically ineffective or unnecessary. In spite of this, the effects of charges on general health status during the term of the experiment were found to be relatively minor (Brook et al, 1983) although this study has been criticised for the use of very limited measures of health status (Donaldson and Gerard, 1989).

Overall it seems unlikely that any significant efficiency gains will be achieved by the new charging regime, not the least because it is secondary services where charges have generally increased and these are less responsive to price than primary health services. Some efficiencies may be achieved if the inappropriate use of hospital services for minor ailments is discouraged. However there is unlikely to be any significant shift towards primary care as long as charges for GP consultations remain as much as, or more, than out-patient hospital charges.

Reducing government expenditure

The primary objective of user charges is usually cost containment. However, although user charges may have had some marginal impact, the levelling off of health care expenditures in other countries in recent years has generally been attributed to other changes in health policy. While the USA has by far the highest user charges, it has had little success in containing health expenditure. As Creese (1991) has noted: "Reforms of most western countries do not appear to centre on a move to greater reliance on direct user charges".

In New Zealand, cost escalation has not been a problem in the past, especially for hospital services. Government per capita expenditure on health actually fell by almost 7% in each of the 2 years preceding the introduction of the new regime. This may be due in part to the use of user charges which had already increased from 13.8% of total health expenditure in 1989 to 18% in 1991 (Muthumala and McKendry, 1991).

The government made it clear that the new regime of user charges is not expected to achieve significant fiscal savings. Nevertheless, budget forecasts for the first year indicate that savings amounting to $95m were expected initially. This official estimate has subsequently been revised downwards several times and, by October 1992, stood at only $32.3m. It now seems likely that few, if any, savings will be achieved, at least in the first year when set-up costs have been high. In part this may be due to poor forecasting and the absence of information about health service utilisation rates by the different income groups. However there has also been widespread resistance to the payment of hospital charges. By the end of the first quarter (May 1992), outstanding debts fell in the range of 30-60% of total revenue from the charges (New Zealand Herald, 1992). This may be an aberration as people become used to the charges and debt collecting procedures are put into place. Unfortunately, as the New Zealand health system is now being restructured and hospitals are becoming more competitive, revenue information is no longer available as it is regarded as "commercially sensitive".

CONCLUSION

The Interim Targeting Regime of user charges recently introduced into New Zealand may improve access to primary care for those in the lowest income groups. But rather than being removed, initial indications are that problems of access have simply been shifted slightly higher up the income scale. Furthermore it seems unlikely that the new regime will make any major contribution towards the other objectives of reducing cost-shifting, improving efficiency through reduced service use, or reducing government expenditure. It is however early days and as yet no firm empirical evidence is available to either prove or disprove the points discussed in this paper.

The introduction of the new regime, especially the introduction of hospital charges, has stimulated widespread debate about appropriate funding mechanisms for health services. While the incumbent (conservative) government has made clear its commitment to user charges, the two main opposition parties have both stated their intention to remove the hospital charges should they be elected to power at the end of 1993. Those in favour of the charges point to the long history of user charges for primary services in New Zealand and the potential inefficiencies in service use when health care is provided free of out-of-pocket charges. Opponents of the new regime tend to focus on the hospital charges, especially their high administration costs and poor revenue.

The Interim Targeting Regime is one part of a much wider reform of the public health system in New Zealand. The debate over user charges has tended to overshadow other elements of the reforms which have greater potential to improve efficiency of resource use.

REFERENCES

Brook, R.H. Ware, J.E., Rogers, W.H. et al (1983), Does Free Care Improve Adults Health? Results from a Randomised Controlled Trial, *New England Journal of Medicine*, 309: 1426-1434.

Creese, A. L. (1991) User Charges for Health Care: a Review of Recent Experience, *Health Policy and Planning*, 6(4): 309-319.

Donaldson, C. and Gerard, K. (1989), Countering Moral Hazard in Public and Private Health Care systems: A Review of Recent Evidence, *Journal of Social Policy,* 18(2): 235-251.

Lohr, K.N., Brook, R.H., Kamberg, C.J. et al. (1986), Use of Medical Care in the Rand Health Insurance Experiment: Diagnosis and Service - Specific Analyses in a Randomised Controlled Trial, *Medical Care,* 24(9), Supplement.

Muthumala, D. and McKendry, C. (1991), *Health Expenditure Trends in New Zealand 1980-1991*, Department of Health, Wellington.

New Zealand Herald, June 18, 1992, *Hospital Fees Unpaid by up to 63pc.*

Shipley, J. (1991) *Social Assistance: Welfare That Works,* Government Printer, Wellington.

Upton, S. (1991) *Your Health and the Public Health: A Statement of Government Health Policy,* Government Printer, Wellington.

Van de Ven, W .P.M.M. (1983), Effects of Cost-Sharing in Health Care, *Effective Health Care* 1(1): 47-56.

Wellington Health Action Committee (1992) *Health Reforms: A Second Opinion.*

3 The Design of a Regional Care Delivery Plan as a Result of Cooperation Among Health Insurers, Health Care Suppliers and Local Government

MARTIEN H. VAN TITS[1] & WIM J. NUIJENS[2]

[1]Tilburg University, The Netherlands
[2]Association of Dutch Sick Funds, The Netherlands

HEALTH CARE REFORMS IN THE NETHERLANDS

The Dutch health care system is in transition. After the publication in 1987 of the so called Dekker-report and the government paper "Change assured", many reforms have either been implemented or are on the drawing board. Overall strategy is aimed at streamlining and improving the traditional "Bismarckian" social insurance system by giving financial incentives to the social insurers in an environment of regulated competition[1].

During the seventies and eighties there emerged concerns that the growing role of government planning and price control had seriously eroded the responsibilities of social insurers and care suppliers. The political climate was ripe for proposals to reduce the influence of the central bureaucracy in order to promote decentralisation of decision making and self regulation by the parties involved. In spite of warnings about overconfidence in market forces, most political parties were optimistic and prepared to go ahead with regulated competition.

A serious complication is the existance of four insurance systems in the Netherlands. These are:

- A general insurance system (AWBZ) covering long term care such as care for physically and mentally handicapped, nursing homes and home care.

---

[1]   For a comprehensive survey of the reforms see: Van de Ven, W. "The key role of health insurance in al cost-effective health care system", Health Policy, 7, 1987, 253 -272

Strategic Issues in Health Care Management. Edited by M. Malek, J. Rasquinha and P. Vacani
© 1993 John Wiley & Sons Ltd

- A sick fund system covering acute illnesses, with rather generous benefits and including about 62% of the population.
- A private insurance system (34% of the population).
- A collective civil servant's insurance system (4% of the population).

To attain a universal and integrated system in which insurers are able to compete, steps have been taken to implement:

- a basic insurance for the whole population.
- freedom to select a health insurer.
- introduction of budgetting methods to allocate centrally collected income dependent premiums among the admitted health insurers (both sick funds and private insurers) according to need-based criteria.
- more freedom for care suppliers and insurers to make contracts regarding the content, quantity and quality of the health services.

Because health insurers cannot cover all their expenses by the contribution from the central fund, they must charge a per capita premium. This is supposed to act as an incentive for cost containment and quality control. This so called nominal premium is to be collected by the insurer directly from its insured persons.

Although these changes involve both severe technical complications and radical institutional rearrangements, the process was continued by the new centre-left government, which replaced the centre-right government in 1990. However at this moment there is a serious deadlock caused by resistance from many sides. Hope remains that the half-way reforms, that bring the worst of both worlds, will be complemented by further changes and reform, such as the necessary integration of the diverse insurance systems[2]. Problems over relative shares of income-dependant and nominal (per capita) premiums continually casts shadows over the proposals that are suggested. Nevertheless no suitable alternatives have been made, although a more cautious approach, aimed at maintaining more government involvement in some sectors, is supported by some opinion leaders. The question of how to budget the insurers, in order to prevent adverse selection and to stimulate good quality of care has not been solved satisfactorily. Continuous strengthening of the position of health insurers, whatever the eventual details of the rules governing the system seems likely. The point of no return appears to have been passed.

THE NEED FOR LONG TERM PLANNING

It is obvious that the increasing responsibility of the health insurers for the quality and cost of health care has implications for their behaviour concerning the hospital planning process.

---

[2]   See: Nuijens, W. "The collectivisation of health insurance", Social Science and Medicine, vol 34, no 9, pp 1049 - 1055, 1992

Here an unexpected paradox appears. In the past sick funds were concentrated in one or two specific districts (operational areas). Even a number of private insurance companies, especially those that were connected to sick funds, concentrated their activities on a geographical basis. Because of the freedom to choose an insurer, the government has drawn up the regional anchor of these insurers and has more or less forced them to work nation-wide.

The supply of care, however, is inevitably organized on a regional level, at least for the basic services. This means that negotiations must take into account local variations and make plans that are designed to cope with the existing needs and available services. This is especially true for investment decisions, because they determine the medical infrastructure for decades to come. This planning process was (and still is) in the hands of the governement, but the declared policy is to bring it back to the "market". However, if there are no insurers with a substantial market share, nobody has reason to be interested, or prepared to engage themselves, in the coordination of local suppliers on such an intensive scale that is relevant for the price and quality of the health care providers. Conversely, an individual professional or even a hospital cannot be expected to deal with a great number of insurers, at least in a way that has meaning for suitably organising health care delivery. At the same time, commercial banks are reluctant to give credit to hospitals or private practices that cannot show that they will have a sufficient number of insurers as contract partners.

Perhaps this paradox will be resolved by the current process of merging insurers. It seems probable that a limited number of big conglomerates will eventually dominate the national market. This implies that oligopoly not perfect competition will be the dominant market form. At the local level, the supplier will then have to make arrangements with, at most, a handful of insurers. This situation is also more suitable to the natural monopolies that exist in health care.

Whatever lies ahead, the local sick fund that dominated the Breda area has decided that a wait and see attitude is not the right policy. Even before the Dekker reforms started, the sick fund had initiated the development of a model that calculates the effect of a substantial reduction of hospital beds on other care suppliers, both institutions and self employed professionals. It was already clear that there were a substantial number of patients present in hospitals that really belonged in nursing homes or homes for the elderly with some additional services. The substitution of services is of prime interest, especially if it leads to better quality and lower costs. Substitution can mean both the replacement of specific services by other services and the replacement of specific professionals by other professionals (or even informal care). The distinction is not always clear cut, as for example the substitution of a medical specialist by a general practioner. It can be argued that GP services are a different form of health care, but the rational that the GP delivers the same services (check ups, prescription of medicine, etc.) but in a different setting is also plausible.

QUANTITATIVE RESEARCH AND A CALCULATION MODEL FOR THE EFFECTS OF CARE SUBSTITUTION

In the Netherlands the government, according to the rules laid down in the Hospital Planning Law, has given permission to the Breda area in the province of North Brabant (390,000 people), to build a new hospital, to extend another and to close one. These hospital planning activities are carried out in combination with a huge bed reduction programme. About 16% of the capacity of hospital beds in the area wil be closed. For this reason the dominant sick fund (AZWZ Breda) has initiated the development of a model that calculates the effects of substitution of care by different institutions and self-employed professionals. Assuming a substantial reduction of the number of hospital beds, the question of what provisions would be necessary, needed to be addressed.   In this light the Institute of Social Research IVA-Tilburg, was asked to carry out the necessary research activities.

The study includes three parts. The first part is a study of the use of hospital care in relation to its necessity.   The research investigates the possible alternatives for hospital care: how much hospital care can be substituted and by what kind of care. The resultant data is used in the second part, to make an integral calculation of the possible outcomes of the bed reduction, in terms of places in nursing homes and homes for elderly, and in terms of manpower: home help, home nursing, general practitioners, self care and informal care. Relations were brought together in a 'substitution matrix' and some versions about substitution possibilities of other care institutions. In the third part, the consequences of bed reduction in general hospitals were studied in combination with the capacity in the present and the future situation of the other care institutions in the area. Bottlenecks are determined and solutions are proposed.

Alternatives for hospital care

Prior to the bed reduction an assessment was made of the number of hospital days which were unnecessarily spent in the general hospital. Twice a day over two weeks, all patients staying in the general hospital to be closed were recorded.

During this period for each patient it was determined if the patient strictly needed to be an in-patient in the general hospital from the medical and from the nursing point of view. The nursing information was supplied by the head of the hospital-ward where the patient was staying and the medical information was given by the medical specialist.

For those patients whose in-patient stay in the general hospital was not strictly necessary for nursing and medical reasons, the best alternative was determined. As all data are collected every day, the results are in terms of "days" and not in terms of "numbers of patients". Table 1 shows the main results.

In 20% of the registered hospital days there appears no strict need for patients to be hospitalized. Self care and informal care seem to be the best alternative for 6% of the in-patient hospital days. Other important alternatives are a somatic nursing home

Table 1. Alternatives for Hospital Care

Alternative	Percentage of Hospital days
General Hospital; day surgery	1.4 %
General hospital; out-patient department	1.4%
Psychiatric hospital	0.6%
Other hospitals	0.2%
Somatic nursing home	4.6%
Psychogeriatric nursing home	0.6%
Home for the Elderly	3.0%
General practitioner	0.4%
Home nursing	0.8%
Home help	0.8%
Sheltered homes for psychiatric patients	0.2%
Self care and informal care	6.0%
Total	20.0%

(4.6%), a home for elderly (3.0%), day surgery in a general hospital (1.4%) and the out-patient department of a general hospital.

Although 20% is a high rate, it must be remembered that this percentage relates to days and not to patients. When a patient, for instance, is staying five days in hospital, then it is possible that the patient's stay in the hospital is not strictly necessary during the first or the last day. In other words: this rate does not mean that 20% of the patients do not strictly need to be in hospital.

Another result of the study is that about 40% of these days cannot be realised, because the patient is on a waiting list for the alternative institution.

Four versions to calculate the results in the middle to long term

Version 1

- the analyses found a total of 20% of the hospital days which could ideally be substituted. The ideal is where there are no waiting lists, the patient does not have any resistance against going home earlier than expected, and where in the home situation there exists sufficient informal help But perfect situations under all circumstances are an illusion. Therefore our basic assumption are:
- that it must be possible to substitute 10% of the hospital days. (It is a fact that 16% of the bed capacity in general hospitals will be closed. We assume that for 6% of the capacity reduction a solution can be found in a more effective way of working. This means that the remaining 10% must be found in substitution).
- that the substitution of these 10% of the hospital days will be by the alternatives found in the first study (table 1), in the same ratio.

Version 2

In the second version our assumptions for in-patient general hospital care are the same as in the version 1. An additional assumption is that almost all different institutions and self-employed professionals can also substitute a part of their care. Substitution takes place from a higher to a lower level; this means for instance that a general practitioner can be a substitute for hospital care, but the opposite situation is not possible.

The substitution rates can be found in table 2. As the care suppliers are arranged from high leveled to low leveled, the upper right half of the substitution matrix is filled.

In the first row of the matrix we find the substitution possibilities for in-patient general hospital care. The percentages are exact half of those of table 1 (the assumption is that 10% and not 20% of the hospital care can be substituted).

The diagonal shows the supposed substitution percentages. In each row we can find the substitutes in their proportions. In case of homes for elderly is, for instance, a substitution possibility supposed of 10%. The substitute is home help (6%) and self care/informal care (4%).

The maximum substitution rate is 10%. This rate we assume for in-patient general hospital care, out-patient general hospital care, somatic nursing homes and homes for elderly. 5% substitution is assumed for the day surgery department of general hospitals, other hospitals and psychiatric hospitals, general practitioners, home nursing and home help. No substitution possibilities are supposed to be in psychogeriatric nursing homes, sheltered homes for psychiatric patients and with self care and informal care.

Here, care in the home situation is accentuated. The difference between version 2 and 3 are the following substitution rates: in-patient department general hospitals 22%, other hospitals 11%, somatic nursing homes 16% and homes for elderly 16%.

For each version a calculation is made to determine the effects for the next five years for all health care suppliers. This is performed by taking demographic developments into account. In order to compare the results, calculations for a basic version were also made. Version zero consists of the growth in use of health care as a result of expected demographic developments; the assumption being there is no substitution. Summarizing, we have the next versions:

version 0	Demographic developments; no substitution;
version 1	Demographic developments and substitution of 10% of in patient general hospital care;
version 2	Demographic developments and substitution with a maximum of 10% for all health care suppliers.;
version 3	Demographic developments and care in the home situation accentuated.

Table 2. Substitution Matrix Version 2 (percentages)

From \ To	Genr Hosp In Pat	GenH Day Surg	GenH Out pat Dep.	Oth Hosp	Psy. Hosp	Somat Nurs. Home	Psy Ger N.H	Home for Eld.	Gen Prac	Home Nur-sing	Home Help	She Hom Psy	Self/ Inf Care
General Hosp. In-Pat.	-10.0	0.7	0.7	0.1	0.3	2.3	0.3	1.5	0.2	0.4	0.4	0.1	3.0
GenHosp Day Surgery		-5.0	5.0	-	-	-	-	-	-	-	-	-	-
GenHosp OutPat Department			-10.0	-	-	-	-	-	8.0	-	-	-	2.0
Other Hospitals				-5.0	-	-	-	-	-	1.0	1.0	-	3.0
Psych Hospitals					-5.0	-	-	-	-	-	-	3.0	2.0
Somatic NursHom						-10.0	-	5.0	-	2.0	3.0	-	-
Psy. Ger NursHom							X	-	-	-	-	-	-
Home for Elderly								-10.0	-	-	6.0	-	4.0
General Practitioner									-5.0	-	-	-	5.0
Home Nursing										-5.0	3.0	-	2.0
Home Help											-5.0	-	5.0
Shelt. Homes Psych.Pat												X	-
Self care and Informcare													X

Where a somatic nursing home is a substitute for in-patient hospital care, then one day will be substituted by another day. The units of measurement are the same. If in-patient days in general hospitals are substituted by out-patient activities in general hospitals, we must transform days into visits; the units of measurements differ. In table 3 we can find the used transformations, only for those substitution situations in which units of measurements differ.

Table 3. Transformations

From	To	Substitution	Substitute
General Hospital In-patient Depart.	General Hospital day surgery	5 days	1 day surg. 3 visits
General Hospital In-patient Depart.	General hospital out-pat. department	3 days	3 visits
General Hospital In-patient Depart.	General practitioner	1 day	3 contacts
General Hospital In-patient Depart.	Home nursing	1 day	6 contacts
General Hospital In-patient Depart.	Home help	1 day	3 contacts
General hospital day surgery	General hospital out-pat. department	1 day surgery	3 visits
General hospital out-patient depart.	General practitioner	1 visit	2 contacts
General hospital out-patient depart.	Self care and informal care	1 visit	1 day
Other hospitals	Home nursing	1 day	6 contacts
Other hospitals	Home help	1 day	3 contacts
Somatic nurs. home	Home nursing	1 day	6 contacts
Somatic nurs. home	Home help	1 day	3 contacts
Home for elderly	Home help	1 day	1 contact
General practitioner	Self and informal care	1 contact	1 day
Home nursing	Home help	3 contacts	1 contact
Home nursing	Self and informal care	1 contact	1 day
Home help	Self and informal care	1 contact	1 day

Table 4 shows the main results of each version. The results are given in mutation percentages in the middle to long term (5 years), in relation to the present.

Version 0 shows how many percentage each health care supplier needs to grow within 5 years, only to cover demografic developments. The highest grow rates are with nursing homes (12.6%) and homes for elderly (14.8%).

If 10% of in-patient general hospital care is substituted, accounting for demographic developments, somatic nursing home capacity needs to grow by 17.2% and the capacity in homes for the elderly by 15.5%. Where all care suppliers have the possibility of substitution (version 2), both the capacity of home nursing and of home help needs to increase by: 13.3% and 17.0% respectively. In the case of strong substitution with in-patient care suppliers (version 2), the number of home nurses needs to increase by 21.6% and the number of home helpers by 27.0%.Consequences of the bed reduction

A general overview of the capacity consequences in the present situation and in the projected situation five years hence for each version was made. Table 5 shows these results. Regarding for the elderly, it appears that the number of beds in the present situation is 2.767. Because of demographic developments (version 0), the capacity should increase to 3.177 beds. Because of the substitution of general hospital capacity (version 1), the number should increase to 3.197 places. If houses for the elderly can substitute 10% of their capacity, the number of places must be 2.910.If all in-patient care suppliers can substitute strongly (version 3), the capacity in houses for the elderly can even decrease a little: from 2.767 places to 2.756 places after 5 years.

Table 4: Main results per version (percentages)

	Version 0 **Demographic developments and no care substitution**	*Version 1* **Demographic developments and substitution of 10% of in-patient gen. hospital care**	*Version2* **Demographic developments and substitution for all care suppliers with a max. of 10%**	*Version 3* **Demographic developments and strong substitution of in-patient care**
General hospital in-patient depart.	+4.1%	-6.3%	-6.3%	**-18.8%**
General hospital day surgery	+4.1%	**+11.1%**	+5.6%	**+13.6%**
General hospital out-patient depart.	+4.1%	+5.0%	-5.2%	-4.2%
Other hospitals	+2.5%	+3.6%	-1.6%	-6.7%
Pshychiatric hosp.	+2.5%	+3.1%	-2.1%	-1.5%
Somatic nurs. home	**+12.6%**	**+17.2%**	+5.5%	+3.2%
Psychoger. nurs. home	**+12.6%**	+13.5%	+13.5%	+14.6%
Home for elderly	**+14.8%**	**+15.5%**	+5.1	-0.4%
General practitioner	+3.0%	+3.2%	+4.0%	+4.2%
Home nursing	+7.7%	**+10.7%**	**+13.3%**	**+21.6%**
Home help	+8.3%	+9.1%	**+17.0%**	**+27.0%**
Sheltered homes for psychiatr patients	+2.5%	+4.8%	**+29.8%**	**+32.7%**
self/informal care	Unknown	Unknown	Unknown	Unknown

Table 5. Capacity consequences per version

Health care supplier	Present situation	Situation after 5 years			
		Version 0	Version 1	Version 2	Version 3
General hospital in-patient depart.	1.486 beds	1.546 beds	1.392 beds	1.392 beds	1.207 beds
General hospital day surgery	7.732 day surg.	8.046 day surg.	8.593 day surg.	8.163 day surg.	8.787 day surg.
General hospital out-patient depart.	486.000 visits	506.000 visits	511.000 visits	461.000 visits	466.000 visits
Other hospitals	282 beds	286 beds	287 beds	280 beds	274 beds
Psyciatric hosp.	346 beds	364 beds	368 beds	332 beds	336 beds
Somatic nurs. home	619 beds	697 beds	726 beds	654 beds	639 beds
Psychoger. nurs. home	375 beds	423 beds	426 beds	426 beds	430 beds
Home for elderly	2.767 beds	3.177 places	3.197 places	2.910 places	2.756 places
General practitioner (full-time working)	159 persons	164 persons	165 persons	166 persons	166 persons
Home nursing (full-time working)	149 persons	161 persons	165 persons	169 persons	182 persons
Home help (full-time working)	719 persons	779 persons	785 persons	842 persons	914 persons
Sheltered homes for psyciatr. patients	69 places	71 places	73 places	90 places	92 places

Comparing the present situation with the situation after 5 years according to version 3 for home nurses and home helpers, a growth is necessary from 149 to 182 persons and from 719 to 914 persons respectively.

Table 5, also shows the difference in capacity consequences between version 1 (demographic developments and substitution of 10% of in-patient general hospital care) and version 0 (only demographic developments). The difference between these two versions is the pure theoretical substitution effect of bed reduction in general hospitals. This means that 154 beds in general hopspitals (1.546 minus 1.392) are substituted by:

- 547 days of day-surgery in general hospitals;
- 5.000 out-patient visits in general hospitals;
- 1 bed in another hospital;
- 4 beds in psychiatric hospitals;
- 29 beds in somatic nursing homes;
- 3 beds in psychogeriatric nursing homes;
- 20 places in homes for elderly;

- 1 general practitioner (full-time);
- 4 home nurses (full-time);
- 6 home helpers (full-time);
- 2 places in sheltered homes for psychiatric patients;
- 12,000 days of self care and informal care.

CAPACITY PLANNING

For the development of a health care plan for the region, not only hospital substitution and demographic trends are of interest. Effects of shortcomings in some provisions, effects of intended expanding activities and waiting lists need to be quantified. The results of this analysis are a prognosis of the future need of care for the Breda area and better insight into the present and future bottlenecks in health care. This important information is provided to enable the sick fund to support its contract policy.

The four most important bottlenecks for the Breda region are: care for elderly, for psychiatric patients, for mentally handicapped and informal care. Initiatives have been taken to resolve these problems. The shortage of somatic and psychogeriatric nursing homes will be relieved by expanding homes for elderly with new wards for these specific categories of patients. Also more specific care in the home situation will be given, in order to facilitate non residential care. Psychiatric patients and mentally handicapped special programs will be developed in order to stimulate them to stay at home for a longer period.

These initiatives, in combination with the fact that hospital substitution generates a need for about 12,000 days self care and informal care, have induced the sick fund to start a research programme for the promotion of informal care. Attention will be focussed on the effectiveness of measures to support family members and volunteers. Without the mobilisation of informal care the possibilities for home care and self care are restricted.

ADDITIONAL MEASURES — INTAKE, INDICATION, AUTHORISATION

Capacity planning is only part of the activities that are necessary to improve the relationship between inputs and outcomes. The insurer should also promote the optimal use of the available facilities, given their availability in the short run.

At this moment the requirements that must be fulfilled in order to receive care covered by legal insurance are diverse. Admittance to a nursing home or to a home for the elderly is only possible after the approval of a municipal indication commission. For hospital treatment, authorisation by the sick fund is a condition, but this is a formality. For specialist treatment a referral by a general practitioner is needed. The situation for home care and medical aids and appliances is even more complicated. Private insurance restrictions depend on the policy chosen by the insured, but are more and more comparable to the sick fund rules.

The financing of the different types of care is not uniform. Nursing homes and the delivery of home care are part of the AWBZ insurance. This is not the case for services like meals on wheels, technical provision like alarm, wheelchairs and lifts, which are, in some cases, covered by the disability insurance. Long term stay in homes for the elderly is, for many people, only possible with social assistance. Costs are controlled by the provinces. It goes without saying that this fragmentation does not favour an efficient use of the existing facilities.

CONCLUSION

The sick fund has proposed a cooperation with the local governments in the Breda area for the establishment of an indication and coordination system. This will eventually lead to a lesser degree of autonomy of the health care sector (especially nursing homes and home care organisations) and the municipalities (especially concerning decisions about social services, home adaptations, transport facilities). This will not be realised without considerable resistance. The aim is not to create one institution with a centralised bureaucracy. Local variations, even in a small and densely populated district, must be taken into account.

Section II

Resource Planning

4 Health Care Delivery Efficiency Indices for Developing Countries — The Search for the Holy Grail

MO MALEK[1], JOE RASQUINHA[1], PAUL VACANI[2&1] & CHRIS EVANS[1]

[1]*University of St Andrews*
[2]*University of Dundee*

INTRODUCTION

Developing countries face a diverse range of developmental objectives and continually attempt to juggle their limited available resources to meet such shifting needs. Health care has received a significant portion of those resources. Because of health cares' uniqueness as a product its continual provision has been viewed as a vital necessity to the community at large, and cost-effectiveness has not played a significant part in the allocation mechanism. In addition, measuring cost-effectiveness in health is difficult, and contemporary measures are woefully inadequate. Even recent innovative efficiency measurement techniques do not portray the whole picture and are at best partial measures of efficiency for policy formulation. Developing countries have come to realise that the granting of *carte blanche* to expenditure in health care is inadvisable. This is because resources are scarce, and health sectors in many developing countries are more concerned with the general improved health status than cost effectiveness of the programmes. Policy makers need better measures to analyse the performance of the health sector as a unit.

This paper evaluates the current popular techniques used to measure, evaluate and base decisions about a country's health care system. The fundamental weaknesses are pinpointed. Attention then turns to appraising alternative existing measurement techniques. These are discussed and again found wanting. In light of this, the paper examines the case for the development of a new cross-country method of evaluation and application: the Healthcare Delivery Efficiency Index (*HDEI* thereafter). The characteristics that ideally should contribute towards such a measure are identified and discussed and a framework for evaluation is suggested.

Strategic Issues in Health Care Management. Edited by M. Malek, J. Rasquinha and P. Vacani
© 1993 John Wiley & Sons Ltd

SOCIETAL HEALTH STATUS PROFILE

It is commonly believed that there is a positive correlation between the stage of economic development and the health profile of a nation, i.e. the more developed nations are, the more healthier they are. The measure of economic development is usually proxied by per capita GDP, an approximation which has always been somewhat controversial in mainstream economics. Since there is also a positive correlation between GDP per capita and the health care expenditure ratio (*HCE* ratio as a percentage of GDP), it is usually argued that social health status can be inferred from the corresponding *HCE* ratios. What is lost in this line of argument is that no allowance is being made for efficiency improvements or better utilisation of resources or what is generally thought of as an increased productivity in economic terms.

In reality, *HCE* ratios are only measures of 'affordability', no more, no less. In economic terms they constitute 'budget constraint's and at best can be thought of as measures of political willingness. This confusion over what is a measure of 'input' and what could at best partially be construed as a measure of 'output', is abundant not only in academic literature, but perhaps more dangerously by the practitioners in the developing countries.

The evidence is available in Appendix 1. This lists an indicative cross section of the various health statistics provided by various international institutions. In spite of their contributions as individual elements to assist policy makers, the measures do not provide an overall picture of the health system nor its managerial and/or its organisational efficiency. Physicians, dentists, pharmacists, nursing personnel and midwifery personnel are necessary for a health system, but they constitute only part of what at best can be called 'inputs', and the present trends amongst developing countries towards increasing their stock *per se* may not be the ideal strategy to pursue for improving health care efficiency (see Malek 1991). Medical personnel are only one element in a health system, albeit an important one. If the system is inefficient, or it does not deliver health care effectively, such personnel tend to emigrate, or concentrate in urban areas or in areas of affluence which provide them with financial security and scope for promotion.

Similarly, health care may be effectively delivered by increased hospital beds, health posts, family welfare centres, health complexes, village health workers, or through efficient immunization programmes, ante-natal care, de-worming, blindness prevention or nutrition services. Yet, although each individual element (input) may contribute positively to the overall output of the health system (the minimum, or the necessary condition), its best use can only be determined when compared with the alternative uses. The important point to remember is that the *health system* requires more than effective health care delivery or increased medical personnel or hospital beds to render it efficient; it needs increased overall efficiency. In practical terms the efficiency of the use of inputs can be determined only when compared with other alternatives. This is the old concept of 'opportunity cost' which intuitively we all learn early in life but tend to forget later.

Measures such as life expectancy, live births by age, abortions, infant mortality, maternal deaths, causes of death, or government expenditure on health are also measures used by policy makers. These measures have provided information health policy makers can secure on the state and performance of health systems, but they are not sufficient either. Again, they apportion greater importance to *elements* of the health system than to the health system as a *unit*. Contemporary measures of health care are therefore inadequate for system level decision making. However, there do exist other measures which have been more recently developed. It is to these this chapter now turns.

CURRENT HEALTH MEASUREMENT TECHNIQUES

GNP/c has long been criticised as inadequate when evaluating or appraising health care systems. It has remained as the primary basis for comparison due to the lack of suitable alternatives. There have, however, been some brave attempts to improve *GNP* measurements for a better evaluation of development.

Morris (1979) was responsible for the development of the Physical Quality of Life Index (*PQLI*), a consolidated index based upon three measures: life expectancy at age one, infant mortality rates, and, levels of literacy. Each of these indicators were assigned to scales. Countries were ranked on an index based on equal weights of each scale, with their position on the index indicative of their level of development. Morris's *PQLI* generated enormous interest and criticism. It was subject to extensive analysis and criticism from a wide range of researchers like Brodsky (1981), Larson and Wilford (1979a; 1979b; 1980), Larson (1985), Larson (1982; 1986), Mukherjee et al (1979), Ram (1980; 1982), and Vidwans (1985).

The introduction of the Disparity Reduction Rate (*DRR*) as a tool to measure the rate of progress in meeting basic needs was another important contribution. The *DRR* attempts to observe the rate at which the disparity between a country's level of performance in any social indicator and the best performance expected in a future target year (for example 2000 AD) is reduced. The advantage of the *DRR* is its flexibility. It can be applied to individual economic indicators like GNP, life expectancy, or *PQLI*. The latest development in socio-economic indices is the Human Development Index (*HDI*) constructed by the UNDP (1991). The original *HDI* in 1990 merged income, life expectancy, and literacy to give an overall figure and ranking. In a series of refinements in 1991, the *HDI* expanded its base of measurement to include not just adult literacy but also mean years of schooling. Moreover, income beyond the poverty level was considered to make a contribution and was thus given a progressively diminishing weight instead of the previously zero weighting. Further, a separate *HDI* has been prepared for women and men for 30 countries which had sufficient information to indicate gender disparities. In total, the *HDI* appears to be one of the least subjective measures of development and offers some useful techniques which could be utilised in a HDEI.

In conjunction with these socio-economic indices, a substantial number of individual health indices have been developed. Though health indices examining micro-aspects of health status are numerous, those examining macro-aspects of health are few and far between. Adlakha (1972) critically examined the influence of age-mortality patterns of the population (as a variable) in model life tables, to estimate various parameters of mortality of populations in developing countries. Boyle and Torrance (1984) reviewed the procedures necessary in developing a multi-attribute health index for use in population health studies and program evaluations, while Mosley (1983) proposed a model that would better determine factors that cause infant and child mortality.

D'Souza (1989) proposed an index which links mortality levels and cause of death, using illustrations of infant mortality. Fanshel and Bush (1970) suggested that present day indicators - crude death rates, infant mortality, life expectancies, and so on are inadequate measures to determine output of a health system. They argued that actors like the impact of poverty, nutrition, population pressures and others must be taken into consideration. Kaplan, Bush and Berry (1976) offered an 'index of well being', whose most significant factor was a weighted life expectancy. However, this index suffers from the detriment of measuring 'health status' rather than 'health care'.

Larson (1982; 1986) is of the opinion that researchers are reluctant to develop a single health index rather than one which analyses individuals. This is due to the fear that a single index across cross cultural comparisons could be crude and over simplistic. Larson proposes a three part index which measures inputs, outputs, and hospital system variables. This index is intended to be an improvement of individual indices of infant mortality, per capita spending on health care, or other health measures. Le Grand (1987) provided a brief summary of a technique that may be used in international comparisons of inequalities of health using inequality measures such as the Gini coefficient, coefficient of variation, etc. Torrance, Thomas and Sackett (1972) proposed a linear health utility scale that allows assignment of utility values to health states, for any disease or treatment programmes in terms of change it produces in overall health utility. Using algorithms, the model ranks programs by their effectiveness/cost ratios or sorts them into a subset achieving the maximum effectiveness under specific constraints. Vilnius and Dandoy's (1990) attempt to construct a priority rating system incorporating various data sources to quantify disease problems or risk factors. Their model ranks public health issues according to size, urgency, severity of the problem, economic loss, impact on others, effectiveness, acceptability, legality of solutions, and availability of resources.

Thus, though the above mentioned socio-economic and health measures have provided an excellent individual foundation for examining the health system, with the exception of Larson, they do not tackle the health system as a unit. In addition, *they offer a way to measure action taken, but do not offer a way to determine what action is actually needed.*

THE CASE FOR THE CONSTRUCTION OF AN HDEI

The rationale for the construction of an improved method of evaluating health care delivery would be:

- To achieve the optimal use of available resources, through improved allocation and targeting of such resources to where they are most needed and give the best 'value for money'.
- To identify effective (and ineffective) health care delivery methods and procedures within countries, and evaluate their transferability to other countries.
- To enhance the planning, organising and control functions of health care systems; again with the intention of improving resource efficiency.
- To facilitate comparison of achievements by health systems through time and/or across countries.

The development of a methodology for the measurement of a Health Care Delivery Efficiency Index (HDEI) will enable international comparisons of health care delivery to be made at the macro-level. It needs to be emphasised that a HDEI will not directly offer solutions to questions of health care delivery, but will act as an indicator as to where such solutions may be found. To this end, corresponding fieldwork in a cross section sample of developing countries will be essential. These empirical studies will be driven by the results of the methodological work performed. Thus, it is envisaged that a HDEI analysis will not lead to a single academic study, but will evolve as a constant and continual process that is subject to frequent review and re-analysis.

The health system in a country can be categorised into two parts, as indicated in Figure 1, which shows the significant structure of the health care delivery system for a country.

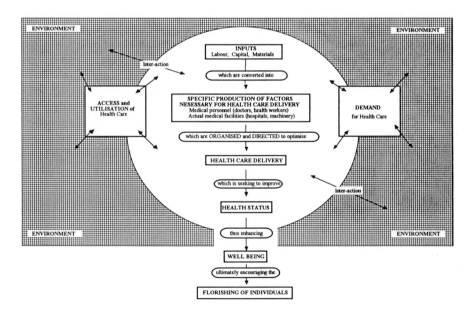

Figure 1. A country's system of health care delivery

Inputs (such as labour, capital, and materials) are combined with the technology to produce intermediate health products.

These interim products are then organised and directed towards selected areas of demand or need in the health care system. They are targeted at the desired final tination of the system: improved health status. Thus in an optimal system, the right mix of the elements of health care will be available in the right place (access) for the right need (demand) to be used (utilised). Environmental factors provide a qualitative background against which the system operates. They consist of culture, policies, fiscal policies, and other factors whose significant influence on health must be recognised, though measurement of these influences may not be directly possible.

A more detailed exposition of the factors requiring evaluation for the construction of an HDEI is schematically represented in Figure 2. The factors include:

-a- **Inputs**
- Labour: consists of direct medical personnel, administrators, managers and others involved in the health system;
- Finance of capital: consists of government expenditure, aid and assistance, and private individuals;
- Materials: includes technology available and physical resources.

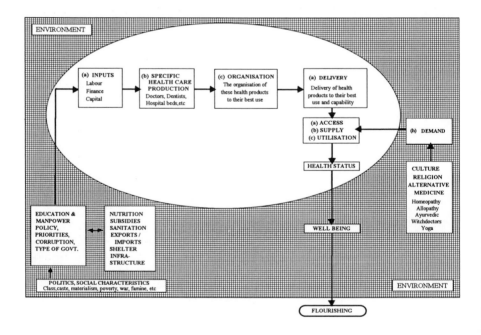

Figure 2. Schematic representation of elements in an HDEI

-b- **Specific health care production** which examines the production of *conventional* health indicators like doctors, dentists, hospital beds, pharmacists, nursing personnel, primary health centres, immunization programmes, village health workers, disease prevention and alleviation programmes.

-c- **Organisation** which analyses the efficiency which conventional health products are organised in the system and identifies bottle-necks.

-d- **Delivery** which observes the delivery mechanism, target population, and the success or failure of the delivery process.

-e- **Access** which analyses the access to health facilities, with consideration to geographical distribution of facilities, topography, cultural and gender bars to access.

-f- **Supply** which caters to the demand conditions, and well as supply conditions in the current system

-g- **Utilisation** which examines the extent to which the health system utilises its facilities (For example, one aspect of utilisation is the degree conventional health indicators like infant mortality, maternity, birth rate, death rate by disease foetal deaths and others have changed, when the health system achieves a higher standard of efficiency).

-h- **Demand** is a significant aspect of the health system. In this analysis, it would include the need or use of alternative forms of medicine like allopathy, homeopathy, the use of indigenous produced medicines, the demand for certain indigenously developed health systems, or the demand for certain aspects of existing health care products.

These factors are essential for the formulation of the *HDEI*. Data is available on most of the variables to ensure a quantitative analysis. However, the influence of what is described in Figure 2 as 'the environment' must be taken into consideration. The *environment* would consist of non-quantitative factors which influence the health system. They can be considered under the following categories:

- Culture and Religion, which have an enormous impact on demand. The wide diversity of developing countries necessitates a brief examination of the effects of culture and religion, which may assist in identifying some of the country-specific influences in the system and the extent to which their influence could be either improved in positive cases, or reduced in negative cases.

- Education and Manpower policies of governments, which include priorities to health and other sectors, their objectives, their will to carry out these objectives, the type of the government in power and the extent of corruption, which will be indicative of their will to implement policy.

- The level of nutrition of the population, sanitation, access to shelter, subsidies of government, import/export performance, infrastructure, and other socio-economic indicators which will indicate the state of the economy.

- Political and social situation of the country, including class, caste, tribal harmony or disharmony, poverty, war, famine, and other variables.

The ideal health system would have an efficient health care delivery and positive environment factors. The methodology of the HDEI will consist of a combination of mathematical and econometric techniques according to the nature of the data, and, parts of established indicators (like the HDI or DRR or other research indices outlined in Section 3 above). All these results will be finally incorporated into a single index to indicate the state of the health system as a whole.

CONCLUSION

Developing an index requires the pin-pointing of the key variables which exert the maximum influence over the system. These key variables are then employed as surrogate representatives of the health care system as a whole. Thus the accurate identification of these key influences within each health care system is crucial. But it needs to be emphasised that any surrogate representative can only do one thing: *represent*. No index can be deemed to be truly interchangeable with the myriad of factors which influence the efficiency of a health care delivery system. Over-emphasis must not be placed on such a representative sets of figures.

Index numbers are merely direction indicators which point to areas worthy of investigation in order to find answers to precise questions. This fundamental failing of index numbers in health care analyses has long been realised by designers of many indices which have been developed for comparative purposes. These have met with differing levels of success, but all have eventually ended in a short life-span and have experienced little lasting acceptance and uptake. In recognising these failings, and through the employment of appropriate steps from the outset to circumvent them, the *HDEI* should prove to be a more robust and substantial analysis; with greater flexibility to cope with divergent and problematic health phenomena, than many previous measures.

This paper has examined some of the major weakness in contemporary methods of health care evaluation and comparison. Reliance upon *GDP* based measures is at best unreliable and may well be highly misleading. There *are* alternative ways of improving health delivery, many of which do not require *GDP* improvements. Admittedly, certain health care improvements can only come about through the introduction of additional resources. However, this injection of funds is not at present our concern.

Properly conceptualized and constructed the *HDEI* will enable field workers to address specific problem countries and provide a commencing point for the study of areas of difficulty. Additionally, the identification of country-specific solutions to individual problems offer scope for utilising such approaches across borders, again offering prospects for improvement of health care delivery. Thus, the successful development of the *HDEI* should shift matters regarding health care delivery further up the international agenda, and hopefully increase the concern for health care problems in developing countries. It may be the case that for the sake of inter-temporal or inter-country comparison such an index is not needed. After all what is really missing is the transferability of the experience of the developing countries in order to prevent repetition of costly and unsuccessful experiments. The fact is the developing countries need to exchange the information. The experience of one country may not be transferable to another geographical and cultural configuration. But, measures of outcome are needed which takes into account special requirement of the developing countries. The real danger is in the absence of such measures. The current controversy regarding outcome measures will be imported to the developing world and given the natural inclination of the 'top' administrators in these countries. One should not be surprised if somebody sooner or later applies QALY's to the developing countries.

ACKNOWLEDGEMENT

The authors wish to thank Catriona Waddington and other participants at the June 1992, Health Economics Study Group Conference, held at the University of St Andrews for their helpful comments and observations.

APPENDIX

Appendix 1   Societal health status measures

TYPE OF MEASURE	UNIT OF MEASUREMENT	AUTHOR / USER
Government Expenditures on health	% of GDP	IMF, Unesco (World Bank (1991))
Dentists	Total Number in Country	U. N. Statistical Yearbook, WHO
Pharmacists	Total Number in Country	U. N. Statistical Yearbook, WHO
Nursing Personnel	Total Number in Country	U. N. Statistical Yearbook, WHO
Midwifery Personnel	Total Number in Country	U. N. Statistical Yearbook, WHO
Hospital Beds	Total number in country	World Health Organisation
Health Posts (each for 6-7000 people)	Total number in country	Choudhury (1981) in OHE (1982)
Family Welfare Centres	Total number in country	Choudhury (1981) in OHE (1982)
Health Complexes	Total number in country	Choudhury (1981) in OHE (1982)
Village Health Workers	Total number in country	Choudhury (1981) in OHE (1982)
Drugs and Biologicals	Availability of 31 essential drugs in public sector, % total requirements	Choudhury (1981) in OHE (1982)
Health Laboratory Services	Simple tests at family welfare centres % coverage	Choudhury (1981) in OHE (1982)
Immunization Against Tuberculoses	% BCG covered children under 15	Choudhury (1981) in OHE (1982)
Control of Tuberculoses	% cases found and treated of estimated total cases	Choudhury (1981) in OHE (1982)
Immunization against diphtheria, Pertussis and Tetanus	% children under 2 immunised	Choudhury (1981) in OHE (1982)

Ante-natal Care	% pregnant women given care at family welfare centres at least once	Choudhury (1981) in OHE (1982)
De-Worming	% children under 15 with worms	Choudhury (1981) in OHE (1982)
Blindness Prevention	% children under 6 receiving vitamin A	Choudhury (1981) in OHE (1982)
Nutrition services	% cases with 2nd and 3rd degree malnutrition found and treated of estimated total cases	Choudhury (1981) in OHE (1982)
AIDS in Developing Countries	HIV infection rate at % of total population	World Bank (1991)
Live Births by Urban/Rural Residence	Total Number in Country and Rates calculated from number of live births / 1000 of population	U.N. Demographic Yearbook
Live Births by age of mother, sex & Urban/Rural Residence	Total Number in Country and Rate	U.N. Demographic Yearbook
Live Birth Rates Specific for age of mother, by Rural/Urban Residence	Rate calculated from live Births by age of mother / 1000 corresponding female population	U.N. Demographic Yearbook
Late Foetal Deaths & ratios by Rural/Urban residence	Total Number & Ratio calculated from foetal deaths / 1000 births	U.N. Demographic Yearbook
Legally induced abortions	Total number in country	U.N. Demographic Yearbook
Legally induced abortions by age & number of previous live births of women	Total number in country	U.N. Demographic Yearbook
Infant deaths and infant mortality rates by age, sex, and Urban/Rural residence	Total number in country & Rate	U.N. Demographic Yearbook
Maternal deaths and maternal mortality rates	Total number in Country	U.N. Demographic Yearbook
Deaths and crude death rates, by Urban/Rural Residence	Total number in country & Rate/number of deaths / 1000	U.N. Demographic Yearbook
Death by age, sex, & Urban/Rural residence	Total number in country	U.N. Demographic Yearbook
Death rates by age, sex & Urban/Rural residence	Rate calculated by number of deaths in age group per 1000	U.N. Demographic Yearbook
Deaths by cause	Total number in country and Rate	U.N. Demographic Yearbook
Expectation of Life by age by sex	Life expectancy calculations	U.N. Demographic Yearbook

REFERENCES

Ahluwalia, M.; Inequality, Poverty and Development. *Journal of Development Economics* 1974: 3, 307-42.

Atkinson, A.; On the measurement of inequality. *Journal of Economic Theory* 1970: 2, 244-63.

Boyle, M.H. and G.W. Torrance; Developing Multi-attribute Health Indexes. *Medical Care* 1984: 22, 11, 1045-57.

Bunge, M.; Development indicators. *Social Indicators Research* 1981: 9, 369-85.

Capozza, D.; An economic index of the quality of life. *Western Economic Journal* 1973: 11, 126.

Choudhury, M.R. (1981), *World Health Forum*, 2, 2,167-73.

Donaldson, C.; Agenda for health: an economic view. *British Medical Journal* 1992: 304, 770-1.

Fanshell, S and J.W. Bush; A health status index and its application to health-services outcomes. *Operations Research* 1970: 18, 1021-66.

Grant, J.P.; 1978: *Disparity Reduction Rates in social indicators: A proposal for measuring and targeting progress in meeting basic needs.* Overseas Development Council, New York.

Jordan, T.; Developing an international index of quality of life for children: the NICQL index. *JRSH* 1983: 4, 127-30.

Koutsoyiannis, A; 1982: *Modern Microeconomics* (second edition). Macmillan, London.

Kravis, I; Z.Kenessy; A.Heston; and R.Summers; 1975: *A system of international comparisons of Gross Product and Purchasing Power.* John Hopkins University Press, Baltimore.

Larson, D.A. and W.T. Wilford; The Physical Quality of Life Index: A useful social indicator? *World Development* 1979: 7, 581-4.

Larson, D.A. and W.T. Wilford; On the Physical Quality of Life Index and evaluating economic welfare between nations. *Economic Letters* 1979: 3, 193-97.

Larson, D.A. and W.T. Wilford; The Physical Quality of Life Index: A new measure of welfare? *Indian Economic Journal* 1980: 27, 3, 53-82.

Larson, D. A test of the stability of the relationship between the Physical quality of Life Index and Gross National Product per Capita. *Indian Economic Journal* 1985: 32, 3, 1-7.

Larson, J.S.; International measures of comparative health care. *Public Health* 1982: 96, 279-87.

Larson, J.S.; A cross-national index of health care. *JHRRA* 1986: Fall, 200-212.

Liser, F.; The measurement of developing progress: a note on the Physical Quality of Life (PQLI) and the Disparity Reduction Rate (DRR). *The United States and World Development Agenda* 1979: 129-44.

Liu, X and J. Wang; An introduction to China's Health Care System. *Journal of Public Health Policy* 1991: 12, 1, 104-16.

Malek, M.; The Impact of Iran's Islamic Revolution on Health Personnel Policy. World Development 1991, 19: 1045-1054

Morris, D.M.; 1979: *Measuring the Condition of the World's Poor: The Physical Quality of Life Index.* Pergamon Press, New York.

Moss, M.; 1973 *The measurement of economic and social performance*. National Bureau of Economic Research; Columbia University Press; New York.

Mukherjee, M.; A.K. Ray and C. Rajyan; Physical Quality of Life Index: some international and Indian applications. *Social Indicators Research* 1979, 6, 283-92.

Newhouse, J.; medical care expenditure: a cross-national survey. *Journal of Human Resources*, 1977: 12, 115-25.

OHE (Office of Health Economics 1982) *Medicines, Health and the Poor World*, 72, April, London: 12 Whitehall (OHE)

Parkin, D.; A. McGuire, and B. Yule; International comparisons of expenditure on health care and its relationship to national income: A critique and some new evidence. 1986: *Health Economics Research Unit*, University of Aberdeen, Discussion Paper 03/86.

Ram, R.; Physical Quality of Life Index and inter-country inequality. *Economic Letters* 1980: 5, 195-99.

Ram, R.; Composite Indices of Physical Quality of Life, basic needs fulfilment and income. *Journal of Development Economics* 1982: 11, 227-47.

Rushingle, E.W.; An economic index of the quality of life. *Western Economic Journal* 1973: 11, 1, 126-127.

Teh-wei Hu; The financing and the economic efficiency of rural health services in the People's Republic of China. *International Journal of Health Services* 1976: 6,2,239-49.

Torrance, G.W.; W.H. Thomas and D.L. Sackett; A utility maximization model for evaluation of health care programs. *Health Services Research* 1972: 7, 118.

UNDP; Human Development Report 1991.

Verhasselt, Y. and B. Mansourian; Method for the classification of countries according to health-related indicators. *Bulletin of the World Health Organization* 1989: 67, 1, 81-4.

Vidwans, S.; A critique of Mukherjee's Index of Physical Quality of Life. *Social Indicators Research* 1985: 17, 127-46.

White, K.L.; Health Surveys: Who, Why and What? *World Health Statistics Health Surveys*. 1985: 38, 1, 2-14.

World Bank (1991), *World Development Report* 1991, New York: Oxford University Press.

5 The SHARP Computer System — A Tool for Resource Planning in the Health Care Sector

FRANK T. DENTON, AMIRAM GAFNI & BYRON G. SPENCER

McMaster University, Canada

INTRODUCTION

Health care absorbs about 7 to 9 percent of the gross domestic product in many developed countries and a substantially higher fraction in the United States.(The Economist) In Canada it accounts for about 9 percent of GDP and represents a continuing source of concern to federal and provincial governments, since much of the cost of providing health care services is met from the public purse. Fuelling this concern is the fact that the population is growing in size, and is also ageing rapidly. Both these issues have important implications for future health care costs. At the same time it has come to be recognized that various institutional arrangements now in place are likely to give providers little incentive to minimize such costs.

The health care system is complex and its evolution can be hard to control. While it can take many years before a decision to train more health care workers has a noticeable effect on the size of the provider stock, once trained such people can remain in the stock for four decades or so, or they can relocate to other jurisdictions in unpredictable ways. Medical technology is advancing rapidly, with major but not necessarily obvious implications for the efficient delivery of services. As the population ages the demands it makes on the system change, but again not in altogether predictable ways: cohort differences in lifestyles, for example, may make health care needs of the next generation of elderly significantly different from those of the current one.

There is universal health insurance in Canada. The operational responsibility for it rests with the Provinces. In addition, each of the ten provincial governments play a major role in determining the number of hospital beds available, the number of applicants who will be accepted into medical schools and nursing programs, the number of hospital positions for interns and residents, and so on. But decisions that are taken regarding one part of the system may ignore repercussions elsewhere; they

Strategic Issues in Health Care Management. Edited by M. Malek, J. Rasquinha and P. Vacani
© 1993 John Wiley & Sons Ltd

run the risk of emphasizing responses to immediate problems while failing to take into account broader and longer-run ramifications. These considerations, and others, provide a strong case for a more systematic approach to planning for the future provision of services.

This paper discusses an integrated set of planning models developed for Ontario, Canada's largest province,[1] and reports some illustrative applications. While the models have been developed for a particular jurisdiction, we believe that the approach has general applicability, and may be of use elsewhere.

AN OVERVIEW OF THE SHARP SYSTEM

SHARP, a System for Health Area Resource Planning, is an integrated set of seven microcomputer-based models.[2]   SHARP has been designed to provide those interested in the health care system with a tool that will help to anticipate problems and a means with which to explore alternative ways to respond to such problems. The first two models of the system project the population to be served and the *requirements* for health care services while the next four project the *availability* of such services. (Projections for up to 50 years are allowed for, although in most applications the period of interest would be no more than a decade or two.) The results are brought together in a *balance evaluation* model, the final one in the system; this model calculates projected imbalances. A user can then explore possible means by which to eliminate or reduce these imbalances.

The system is depicted in broad outline in Figure 1. Rectangles represent the seven individual models and the collection point for information about resource availability; ovals represent parameters to be specified by users. The arrows indicate directions of information flow among the various components.

The **SHARP1** model projects the user population, separately for males and females, by single years of age. The time path of the population is determined by its initial age and sex distribution, the subsequent age-specific rates of fertility and age-sex-specific rates of mortality, the levels and age-sex distributions of foreign immigrants and emigrants, and the levels and distributions of interprovincial migrants.

The requirements for health care services are generated in **SHARP2**.   The fundamental idea here is that the average requirements of each age-sex group for each type of health care service can be specified. Age-utilization profiles have been developed for the requirements for other health care services. The profiles reflect current practice. They are used in SHARP2 to define the default or reference levels of service provision. However, a user need not accept these default profiles: he or she can explore the implications of maintaining current delivery practices (by using the default profiles) or of introducing different practices (by changing the profiles).

---

1   The population of Ontario is about 10 million, out of a total Canadian population of about 27 million.

2   For an earlier report on the SHARP project, see Denton, Gafni and Spencer (1992).

It is emphasized that requirements are defined so as to be entirely independent of the *availability* of services: the requirements change only in response to population change, conditional on the specified utilization profiles. The requirements/availability dichotomy is an essential feature of the SHARP system.

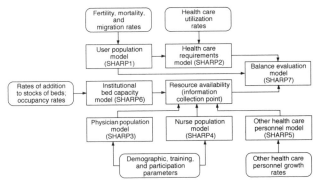

Figure 1: Summary depiction of the SHARP system

SHARP3 and **SHARP4** are concerned with physician and nurse populations, respectively, and with the associated availability of services. Projections are made separately for male and female physicians and nurses, by age. In the case of physicians, SHARP3 keeps separate track of each of thirty specialities. Basic demographic techniques are applied to move the populations forward year by year over the projection period: allowance is made for mortality, migration and retirement; the training of new personnel is taken account with respect to the numbers involved, their age and sex distributions, and the lengths of their training periods; retraining of practising physicians and the associated transfers among specialities are provided for; participation ratios are applied to determine the numbers of full-year equivalent practising personnel, and hence the numbers of person-years of services available.

The supplies of registered nursing assistants and of personnel in 25 other health care worker categories are dealt with in **SHARP5**. The projection procedures are much simpler in this model, requiring only that an overall net rate of growth and a participation ratio be specified for each category.

Institutional bed capacity is modelled in **SHARP6**, which keeps track of the numbers of beds in 11 bed categories and 14 categories of institutions. Starting from the initial stocks, the time paths of the numbers of beds are projected under user-supplied assumptions about net rates of addition to the stocks. Occupancy rates are incorporated as user-supplied input and the numbers of occupied beds calculated so as to allow for normal or assumed underutilization.

The projected requirements and availability of all kinds are brought together in **SHARP7**, the balance evaluation model. Specifically, SHARP7 accepts as input the health care requirements outputs from SHARP2 and the resource availability outputs from SHARP3, SHARP4, SHARP5, and SHARP6. It also accepts population measures from SHARP1 so that ratios of resources to population can be calculated. SHARP 7 displays the imbalances between requirements and availability, and provides related analytical calculations of various kinds. It thus allows a user to determine what changes in rates of addition to personnel populations, institutional bed capacities, or health care delivery practices would be necessary to bring the requirements and availability of different kinds into balance. The balance/imbalance implications of alternative future patterns of health care delivery, medical and nursing school enrolment, etc., can then be studied as a basis for informed policy decision making.

OPERATION OF SHARP AS AN INTEGRATED SYSTEM

The SHARP system is embodied in microcomputer-based software that has been designed to provide a high degree of flexibility and user convenience. The system incorporates a large number of parameters. However, as noted above, default or reference values are supplied in all cases so that a user need change only the particular ones that are of interest in any given application. The software generates some basic output tables but also provides for several hundred optional tables that can be selected by a user who is interested in additional detail. Projections can be made from 1990 or some alternative recent year (again at the option of the user) and can extend up to fifty years. Parameter values can be respecified at points in the projection period to allow for future changes in technology or delivery practices. A user can run the programmes, observe the requirements/availability imbalances, and then re-run it under alternative parameter specifications in order to evaluate the impact of different policy options. Alternative policy options are readily specified in SHARP, and each new projection run takes very little computer time. In consequence, user attention is focused easily and naturally on the practical difficulties of planning in the health care system itself, and not on the technical demands of the models or the software.

A PROJECTION OF HEALTH CARE REQUIREMENTS

Consider first a projection designed to address the question, "How would health care requirements vary if current utilization practices were to be maintained while the population alone changed?" We base such a projection on the use of SHARP1 and SHARP2, in which the underlying parameters of the system are all assigned the reference values. In the case of the population, that means that the total fertility rate remains at its recent level (1.83 births per woman), that mortality rates continue to decline, but somewhat less rapidly than in the last decade or so, and that net immigration into Ontario, from both inside and outside Canada, continues roughly at recent levels. It means also that all utilization profiles remain constant. What would happen to the requirements for health care services in such a case?

Some answers are provided in Table 1, which reports the 1990 population and the associated requirements for selected health care services, together with projections shown in index form at five-year intervals for the next 20 years. For purposes of calibration, the 1990 base period requirements for each type of health care service are set equal to the actual level of service utilization in that year.

The population is projected to grow by 18.9 percent by the year 2000, as compared to 1990, and by 37.3 percent by the year 2010. Focusing on the decade of the 1990s, if current utilization practices were to be maintained, the requirements for health care services would grow more rapidly than the population (the increases are of the order of 20 to 30 percent) as a result of the shifts in age distribution. (The median age of the Ontario population is projected to increase by almost 3 years over the decade.) The biggest increases are for institutional beds, especially those that provide nursing home and residential care (which are in the category 'non-hospital long-term beds') and other forms of what is generally long-term care (those classified as "other hospital beds"; included in this category are general and special rehabilitation, chronic psychiatric, and other chronic care beds).

Table 1. Projected population and health care service requirements
Ontario, 1990-2010 - reference projection

Year	Population	Physician	Interns & Residents	Reg Nurses	Institutional Beds		
					Total	Acute Care	Other Hosp. Beds	Non-hosp. Long-term Beds
Levels								
1990	9,754	17,516	2,957	58,406	125,471	30,643	17,010	77,817
Index								
1990	100.0	100.0	100.0	100.0	100.0	100.0	100.0	100.0
1995	109.7	111.0	112.9	112.7	114.7	112.4	114.7	115.6
2000	118.9	120.9	125.8	124.8	130.7	124.3	130.9	133.2
2005	127.9	131.1	139.7	137.9	148.0	137.2	148.6	152.1
2010	137.3	142.4	155.5	152.6	166.9	151.7	168.9	172.5

Note: With respect to the 1990 levels variables, the population is in thousands, personnel requirements are in full time equivalent person-years, and insititutional beds are in bed year

The growth of requirements in these long-term stay categories exceeds that of the population by more than 60 percent. In SHARP2, the requirements for interns and residents and for hospital-based registered nurses are related to those for institutional beds, by type. The growth in requirements for the services of these groups is somewhat less than for beds, since so much of the increased demand for beds is for long-term stay beds that have relatively low personnel requirements. But it is still substantial more than 30 percent greater than the percentage growth of the population. For physicians the increases are smaller, but nevertheless somewhat greater than the rate of population growth, reflecting the relatively heavy loading of requirements associated with older people for the services of many physician specialities.

How much of the change is due to population ageing and how much to growth? These questions are addressed in the projections reported in the first two panels of Table 2. In the first of these only the size of the population is allowed to increase; its age-sex composition is artificially held constant at the 1990 distribution.[3] The increase in size alone leads to an equal proportionate increase in requirements for each category of health care service, as would be expected. Thus, for example, instead of a 30.7 percent growth in institutional bed requirements by the year 2000, the increase is only 18.9 percent. In the second panel the population size is held constant, but its age-sex distribution is allowed to change year by year as it does in the projection underlying Table 1. Hence there is ageing, but no growth, and the increases in requirements result virtually entirely from changes in the age composition of the population. (The sex distribution is allowed to change also, but that is of negligible importance.) As can be seen from the table, the effects of the compositional changes are substantial, although less than those associated with growth alone.[4] By 2000, ageing alone would increase requirements for institutional beds by 10 percent, and the effects would be greater for long-stay beds. For interns, residents, and for nurses the increases would be smaller, and for physicians, they would be smaller still, less than 2 percent.

SHARP can also be used to isolate the requirements associated with migration. The projection in the last panel of Table 2 is the same as the reference case except that all population movements into and out of Ontario cease; hence all population change after 1990 is the result of natural increase alone. By comparison with Table 1 it can be inferred that in the reference projection less than half of the population growth between 1990 and 2000 is associated with natural increase, more than half with net immigration; by 2010 only about one-third of the growth is attributable to natural increase. As would be expected, then, all increases in requirements are reduced when migration is eliminated. However, the increases in requirements are still relatively greater than the increases in population. The most notable example is again the growth in non-hospital long-term beds, for which the growth in requirements is more than three times the growth in the population by 2000, and more than four times by 2010. This relatively large increase in requirements results from the fact that, given the initial age structure of the population, natural changes alone would lead to a significantly larger proportion of people in the older age groups. (Migrants tend to be more concentrated in the young and middle-age adult years, that is, in age groups that make relatively light demands on health care resources.)

---

3   The population projections that underlie this artificial case and also the next one are of purely analytical interest; they required some supplementary programming outside the main SHARP system.

4   It should be noted that the separate effects of "size" and "ageing" do not sum exactly to the total effect, which includes also the interaction of the two.

Table 2. Indexes of Projected Population and Health Care Service Requirements
Ontario, 1990 -2010 Population Projections of Analytical Interest

Year	Population	Physicians	Interns & Residents	Regis'd Nurses	Institutional Beds			
					Total	Acute Care	Other Hosp. Beds	Non-hosp. Long-term Beds
Only Population Size Changes								
1990	100.0	100.0	100.0	100.0	100.0	100.0	100.0	100.0
1995	109.7	109.7	109.7	109.7	109.7	109.7	109.7	109.7
2000	118.9	118.9	118.9	118.9	118.9	118.9	118.9	118.9
2005	127.9	127.9	127.9	127.9	127.9	127.9	127.9	127.9
2010	137.3	137.3	137.3	137.3	137.3	137.3	137.3	137.3
Only Population Distribution Changes								
1990	100.0	100.0	100.0	100.0	100.0	100.0	100.0	100.0
1995	100.0	101.1	102.9	102.7	104.5	102.5	104.5	105.3
2000	100.0	101.7	105.8	105.0	110.0	104.6	110.1	112.1
2005	100.0	102.5	109.2	107.7	115.7	107.3	116.1	118.9
2010	100.0	103.7	113.2	111.1	121.6	110.5	123.0	125.6
Population Change Reflects Only Natural Increase								
1990	100.0	100.0	100.0	100.0	100.0	100.0	100.0	100.0
1995	106.1	107.7	110.5	110.0	112.6	109.8	112.8	113.7
2000	109.2	112.1	118.9	117.4	124.9	117.0	125.8	127.8
2005	111.3	115.8	127.8	124.9	137.5	124.5	139.3	142.3
2010	112.8	119.7	137.5	133.3	150.7	132.7	154.2	157.0

A PROJECTION OF AVAILABILITY AND RESOURCE IMBALANCES

Projected resource availability in the SHARP system is formally independent of projected requirements. Thus, for example, the physician population, by age, sex, and speciality, and the associated flows of potential health care services, are determined by the migration, retirement, and ageing of physicians and by enrolment in medical schools and intern-residency programs, and *not* by what happens to requirements. It is probably desirable to see a reasonable balance between the future services that will be available, on the one hand, and the future requirements, on the other. The means of achieving a balance are considered and assessed within the SHARP framework through comparisons of projections under alternative assumptions. SHARP thus provides a very inexpensive "laboratory" in which the implications of alternative policy measures can be considered.

Underlying the reference projection of resource availability presented here is the assumption that past practices are continued. In the case of physicians, a constant level of enrolment in medical schools is assumed, together with a constant flow through to the various intern/residency programs (including a net positive intake from out-of-province sources). Upon completion of intern/residency programs, some physicians leave the province to practice elsewhere. We assume that an equal number who have completed similar programs elsewhere enter practice in Ontario, so that the gross addition to the physician stock each year is just equal to the number graduating from the province's intern-residency programs. Enrolment in nursing schools is assumed to grow at 1 percent per year and the net immigration of nurses is set at 1000 per year, or just over 1 percent of the 1990 nurse population. In both cases the enrolment assumptions are consistent with experience over the previous decade; the available data provide less information about the actual movements of physicians and nurses into and out of the province, and the migration assumptions are therefore somewhat more arbitrary.

Recent policy in Ontario has led to a substantial reduction in the overall number of bed days available. For projection purposes we have assumed that the rate of growth of bed days of each type will rise (or the rate of decrease diminish) until it reaches the overall annual rate of population growth, by the year 2000.

Table 3 shows the projected availability (in terms of annual service flows) of each of the same personnel and institutional bed groups identified separately in the previous tables. The services available in 1990 are the same as the 1990 requirements, by assumption, but the projections for subsequent years are independent of requirements. As seen in the table, the population of physicians is projected to increase by about 30 percent by 2000 and 60 percent by 2010. The population of nurses is projected to increase by about 20 percent and 35 percent over the same periods, while for beds, the rates of growth are much slower. The projected 30 percent growth in the availability of physician services is considerably less than what occurred in the period 1980-90, when the overall increase is estimated to have been in excess of 40 percent. The near constancy of projected intern and resident services is roughly consistent with what occurred in the 1980s, as is the 20 percent growth in nursing services.

The imbalances between requirements and availability are shown for the reference projection in the first panel of table 4, where they are expressed as percentages of availability. Each category of service is in balance in 1990, by assumption. In the

Table 3. Projected Health Care Service Availability
Ontario, 1990-2010 -- Reference Projection

Year	Physicians	Interns & Residents	Reg. Nurses	Institutional Beds			
				Total	Acute Care	Other Hosp. Beds	Non-hosp. Long-term Beds
			Levels				
1990	17,516	2,957	58,406	125,471	30,643	17,010	77,817
			Indexes				
1990	100.0	100.0	100.0	100.0	100.0	100.0	100.0
1995	115.3	98.8	110.3	100.9	98.5	100.5	101.9
2000	130.8	98.9	120.0	106.7	104.2	106.3	107.8
2005	145.4	98.9	128.0	114.9	112.1	114.4	116.0
2010	158.9	98.9	134.8	123.5	120.5	123.0	124.8

Note: With respect to the 1990 levels variables, the personnel requirements are in full-time equivalent person-years and institutional beds are in bed-years.

years after 1990, a positive imbalance indicates a surplus, a negative imbalance a deficit. We see that the assumptions result in a projected surplus of physicians of 7.5 percent by 2000 and 10.4 percent by 2010. At the same time, there is a persistent and increasing shortfall in the availability of interns and residents, institutional beds and, to a lesser extent, registered nurses. For interns and residents, the shortfall is 27.2 percent of availability in 2000 and 57.3 in 2010. For institutional beds (all types combined), the corresponding figures are 22.5 and 35.1 percent. The contrast between the physician surpluses and the intern/resident deficits highlights the difficulties that can arise when interns and residents are current service providers as well as the major source of future growth of the physician population.

The imbalances associated with each of the three analytical population projections are displayed in the last three panels of Table 4. Increases in population size alone (with age distribution constant, as in the second panel) cause requirements to increase by less than in the reference case; hence the projected surplus of physician services is increased and the deficits for all other services are reduced. (In the case of nurses the deficits are replaced by small surpluses, prior to 2010.) Ageing alone (the third panel) causes requirements to increase, but at a much slower pace, and the surplus of physicians is thus greater still, and the deficits for other services further reduced (or turned into surpluses). As noted earlier, natural increase, operating in the absence of migration, results in much slower population growth and more rapid ageing than in the reference projection, and in consequence results in a greater surplus of physician services and smaller deficits or modest surpluses for other services.

REDUCING THE IMBALANCES

If the reference projection is accepted as a rough indication of what will happen in the health care system in the absence of changes in policy or practice, the alternative courses of action are clear, in general outline. Projected imbalances could be reduced by modifying either service requirements or resource availability, or both. The particular advantage of the SHARP system is that it helps to focus the discussion of choice and to quantify the implications of alternative actions.

Consider, first, options for altering requirements. In the examples presented, the utilization profiles are held constant over the projection period and that, together with population change, is what gives rise to the increases in requirements. But the utilization profiles in SHARP reflect simply current practice. Perhaps at least some forms of current practice can be changed. Barer and Stoddart (1991: 1-2), in their comprehensive review of the Canadian medical system, have argued that "a non-trivial amount of medical services utilization is ... ineffective, inappropriate, or inefficient". Perhaps one could define some types of current utilization that could be eliminated without adverse health consequences for the population. There is also some scope for modifying service delivery practices to make greater use of less highly qualified personnel, where appropriate for example, through the greater use of nurse practitioners or midwives with concomitant reductions in the requirements for

Table 4. Projected Health Care Service Imbalances as Percent of Availability
Ontario, 1990-2010 — Reference Projection and Projections of Analytical Interest

Year	Physicians	Interns & Residents	Reg Nurses	Institutional Beds			
				Total	Acute Care	Other Hosp. Beds	Non-hosp. Long-term Beds
				Reference Case			
1990	0.0	0.0	0.0	0.0	0.0	0.0	0.0
1995	3.7	-14.3	-2.2	-13.7	-14.2	-14.1	-13.4
2000	7.5	-27.2	-4.0	-22.5	-19.3	-23.1	-23.6
2005	9.8	-41.3	-7.7	-28.9	-22.4	-29.9	-31.1
2010	10.4	-57.3	-13.2	-35.1	-25.9	-37.2	-38.2
				Only Population Size Changes			
1990	0.0	0.0	0.0	0.0	0.0	0.0	0.0
1995	4.8	-11.1	0.5	-8.7	-11.4	-9.2	-7.6
2000	9.1	-20.2	0.9	-11.4	-14.1	-11.8	-10.3
2005	12.0	-29.4	0.0	-11.4	-14.1	-11.8	-10.3
2010	13.6	-38.9	-1.8	-11.2	-13.9	-11.6	-10.0
				Only Population Age Distribution Changes			
1990	0.0	0.0	0.0	0.0	0.0	0.0	0.0
1995	12.3	-4.2	6.9	-3.6	-4.0	-4.0	-3.3
2000	22.2	-7.0	12.5	-3.1	-0.4	-3.6	-4.0
2005	29.5	-10.5	15.8	-0.7	4.3	-1.5	-2.5
2010	34.7	-14.6	17.6	1.6	8.3	0.0	-0.7
				Population Change Reflects Only Natural Increase			
1990	0.0	0.0	0.0	0.0	0.0	0.0	0.0
1995	6.6	-11.8	0.2	-11.6	-11.5	-12.2	-11.5
2000	14.3	-20.3	2.2	-17.0	-12.3	-18.3	-18.6
2005	20.4	-29.2	2.4	-19.7	-11.0	-21.7	-22.6
2010	24.7	-39.1	1.1	-22.0	-10.1	-25.3	-25.8

physician services. (For an analysis of the potential savings associated with greater use of nurse practitioners, see Denton *et al* 1983.) In general terms, the utilization profiles could be redrawn and a plan designed to bring actual profiles into line with the more desirable (less expensive) ones by specified target dates. SHARP could then be used to explore the implications of a gradual transition towards this more effective deployment of health care resources.

Attention could also be focused on ways to increase or reduce resource availability. In the case of a projected shortage of nurses, for example, one could consider policies (perhaps relating to wages or working conditions) designed to reduce the proportion of qualified people who leave nursing well before the conventional age of retirement. Where there are projected surpluses (as in the case of physicians), it is natural to ask whether they might offset projected deficits elsewhere in the system (interns and residents, for example). It may be the projected availability of physicians could be reduced by admitting fewer into medical schools and into intern and residency programs. In this connection Barer and Stoddart (1991: 1-4) recommend that the number entering Canadian medical schools be reduced by somewhat less than 10 percent. (Such a change would, of course, increase the projected shortfall of available intern and resident services; a comprehensive plan would have to take account of that difficulty.) Within the physician population itself, a projected shortage of the services available from one speciality might be offset by reducing surpluses elsewhere for example, by encouraging fewer residents to enter the surplus specialities, or by encouraging those already working in one speciality to consider transferring to another.

CONCLUDING REMARKS

This paper has described and illustrated the use of SHARP, a microcomputer-based system of models developed as a tool to assist health care planners. The SHARP software projects future requirements for health care services in considerable detail while allowing planners to simulate, by computer experiment, the resource implications of alternative patterns of service delivery, resource augmentation, and population growth.

A benefit of the SHARP system is that it focuses attention on projected imbalances between requirements and availability, and on alternative policy initiatives designed to reduce or eliminate the imbalances. Discussions about possible policies or actions are automatically directed to considerations of their implications for resource use in the context of the overall health care system. Another benefit of considerable practical importance is that the development of a system such as SHARP brings to light gaps and weaknesses in the available health care statistics. There is a surprising lack of high quality information in some cases; indeed it was necessary to spend a large portion of the SHARP development time simply piecing together a data base and the initial applications of the system have shown up some of the deficiencies even more clearly. No doubt the availability of information will vary from one jurisdiction to another, but in most jurisdictions there would be considerable benefit from the type of disciplined scrutiny and attempts at integration imposed by working within a comprehensive framework such as the one in which the SHARP system was conceived.

ACKNOWLEDGEMENTS

Project support was provided by the Health Innovation Fund of the Ontario Premier's Council. The research assistance of Christine Feaver, Mark Brockington, Neno Li-Ritchie, and Barbara Markham is gratefully acknowledged.

REFERENCES

Barer, Morris L. and Stoddart, Greg L. (1991), *Toward Integrated Medical Resource Policies for Canada: Background Document*, Centre for Health Economics and Policy Analysis Paper 91-7, McMaster University, Hamilton.

Denton, Frank T., Gafni, Amiram, and Spencer, Byron G. (1992), 'Resource Requirements and Availability: An Integrated System of Models for Health Care Planning', Chytil,

M.K., Duru, G., van Eimeren, W., and Flagle, Ch.D. (eds.), *Health Systems: The Challenge of Change*, Prague: Omnipress, 635 - 638.

Denton, Frank T., Gafni, Amiram, Spencer, Byron G., and Stoddart, Greg L. (1983), `Potential Savings from the Adoption of Nurse Practitioner Technology in the Canadian Health Care System', *Socio-Economic Planning Sciences*, 17 (4), 199-209.

Health Care Survey *The Economist* p 4, July 6, 1991

6 Economic and Health Policy Issues in Biomedical Technology — The Case of Greece

J.E. KYRIOPOULOUS & D.A. NIAKAS

Athens School of Public Health, Greece

INTRODUCTION

Over the last ten years, significant changes have come about in health care services in Greece. The introduction of the National Health System (NHS) in 1983 brought about a huge expansion of the public sector in human, economic and material resources. This development has been accompanied by the extension of health care coverage to the entire population and there has been more equal access to health care provision as well as a more equal distribution of health care resources, at least at the geographical level (Niakas and Kyriopoulos 1992a).

More specifically, during the 1980s despite the recession in the Greek economy, there was a constant increase in health care expenditures. Total health expenditures were increased from 6.5 percent of GDP in 1980 to 8.3 percent in 1990. In particular, according to the National Accounts (OECD data underestimate private expenditures) public health expenditures in the same period rose from 3.8 to 5.3 percent of GDP and private expenditures increased from 2.7 to 3.1 percent respectively (Kyriopoulos 1993). This phenomenon of high increases in health spending in a period of fiscal crisis has been attributed to the introduction of the NHS (Kyriopoulos 1990), the lack of an appropriate and effective method of financing, the absence of cost containment policies (Niakas 1991; Niakas and Kyriopoulos 1992b), and, to the large increases in private diagnostic centres which provide high level medical technology resulting in greater spending. In spite the fact that prices for C-T scanner examinations were constant in the year 1990-91, the total cost was duplicated.[1]

The NHS was established to create a state monopoly, (similar to the British one before the introduction of internal market), and it imposed serious restrictions on the development of the private sector. To succeed in its targets, the Greek NHS law

---

[1] Unpublished data for two main Sickness Funds (IKA and OGA).

Strategic Issues in Health Care Management. Edited by M. Malek, J. Rasquinha and P. Vacani
© 1993 John Wiley & Sons Ltd

prohibited the establishment of new private clinics. At the same time the government kept the reimbursement prices of hospitals from Sickness Funds at low levels, and caused the collapse of many clinics. In this manner, private beds were drastically reduced. Table 1 indicates the development of beds before and after the NHS in both public and private sector.

Table 1. Hospitals and beds before and after the NHS in Greece

	Hospitals		Beds			
	1980	1987	1980 Total number	%	1987 Total number	%
Public	112	136	25905	43.7	35290	68.6
Private	468	267	25075	42.3	15900	30.9
Voluntary non-profit	28	5	8347	14.0	243	0.5
	648	408	59329	100	51443	100

Source: Department of Health Economics, Athens School of Public Health

However, the above restrictions were mainly concerned with the hospital sector. No limits or obstacles were imposed on other areas of provision. For example, the number of doctors entering the profession were increased, and, a number of private health or diagnostic centres were developed (KEPE 1988). These centres mushroomed after 1985 especially in the urban centres (Athens and Thessaloniki). Most of them had introduced high medical equipment and technologies such as Ultrasound, C-T scanners, and Nuclear Magnetic Resonance's (NMRs). Three reasons may explain this quick adaptation in the private sector, especially in Greece. Firstly, the need of the private sector for profits. Secondly, the prices charged for these services of high technology seemed to be higher than the cost of production. And thirdly, the bulk of these services were constantly being increased since any demand of physicians were met without any control by the Sickness Funds or hospitals.

When the conservatives came to office in the beginning of the current decade, the priorities of the national health policy were reversed and there was an attempt to establish a fully competitive market in the health sector. Restrictions on the private sector were removed, and cuts in public spending were intensified. A new Health Law intending to enforce management and create competition among providers was enacted, but there are doubts on its operational capability (Niakas 1992).

INVESTMENTS IN HEALTH AND MEDICAL TECHNOLOGY.

Public and private investment also increased in the last decade. More specifically, public investment increased from 0.08 percent of GDP in 1980 to 0.25 percent in 1991. At the same time private investment increased from 0.04 percent to 0.42 percent over the same period (Kyriopoulos et al 1992). Table 2 indicates the development of public and private investment in health care in Greece in the 1980s. It

Table 2. Time trends of public, private and total health investment in Greece, 1981-1991
(in million drs and current prices)

Year	Public	Private	Total
1981	3857	1740	5597
1982	2697	2431	5128
1983	6055	2239	8294
1984	8689	3668	12357
1985	10979	4823	15802
1986	14867	10526	25393
1987	14403	12000	26403
1988	15236	8845	24081
1989	14310	18916	28266
1990	12734	21007	33761
1991	16314	28103	44417

Source: National Accounts

is worth noting that private investment has increased since 1986, and has in the last three years been overtaking public investment.

The breakdown of investment activity in the public and private sector is also of particular interest. On the one hand in the public sector, investments are evenly distributed, with 50 percent being directed to the purchase of land, buildings and construction, and the remainder being divided between ordinary equipment and medical technology. On the other hand, about 90 percent of private investment is being directed towards high technology. The rapid diffusion of medical technology, especially during the last few years has had a considerable effect on the formulation of national health policy and commitment of resources to other priorities, given that the main volume of investments has occurred in the private sector and in the major urban centres.

Table 3 shows the trends in the development of selective medical technologies in Greece in the public and private sector. The data confirms the rapid growth of private sector especially in C-T scanners and NMRs where opportunity for profit making exists. Further, the public sector is the leader in other technologies such as transplant centres. For example, only last year was a private centre for heart

Table 3. Time trends of biomedical technology in Greece

	1980	1985	1990	1992
CT Scanners	6 (4)	15 (10)	66 (22)	121 (22)
NMRs	-	1	4 (2)	9 (2)
Heart Transplant Centres	-	-	1 (1)	3 (2)
Liver Transplant Centres	-	-	-	1(1)
Kidney Transplant Centres	-	2 (2)	4 (4)	4 (4)
Lithotrepters	-	2 (2)	3 (2)	5 (3)

In brackets the capacity of the public sector
Source: Department of Health Economics, Athens School of Public Health

transplants opened. This was because the Ministry of Health decided to assist in financing these operations in an attempt to limit patients being treated abroad. Of particular interest is a comparison of Greece with the mean average of other countries of the European Community on the use of high medical technologies. Table 4 shows that though Greece has two times more ultra sound equipment and C-T scanners per million inhabitant than other European countries it remains at the same level in comparison with the number of transplant centres. At the same time the number of operations per million inhabitants is much lower in Greece than in other European countries.

The above comparisons lead us to conclude that there is an excess supply of medical technology in Greece in comparison with the EC countries. This excess supply creates the following problems:

• Since the number of produced services is excessive in case of C-T scanners and Ultrasound equipment, there is an over-consumption in health care. This may be attributed either to medical uncertainty or to the complete freedom of Greek physicians to order any expensive diagnostic test even when they are practising at primary health care level and have a first contact with the patient. Alternatively, if the number of produced services is less than the mean average of EC countries, then one may conclude that the productivity in health care in Greece faces serious problems.

• In case of health care transplants performed by the number of operations per million inhabitants, it seems that productivity and efficiency in Greece is lower in comparison with EC countries.

Table 4. High medical technology in Greece and Europe (12) per million/inhabitants.

	Greece (1991)		Europe (1988)	
	Number	Indice	Number	Indice
CT Scanners	12.5	-	5.0	-
Ultrasounds	21.4	-	13.5	-
Lithotrepters	0.50	-	0.88	-
Dialysis	-	390	-	381
Kidney Transplant Centres	0.40	17.1	0.60	26.2
Heart Transplant Centres	0.33	0.6	0.23	5.5
Liver Transplant Centres	0.20	0.2	0.17	3.7

Sources: Figueras et al (1992) and Department of Health Economics,
Athens School of Public Health

It should be noted that a recent study has shown that though current health spending will remain more or less steady throughout the decade of 1991-2000, total investment and, in particular, private investment in high level biomedical technology will rise at a constant rate (Kyriopoulos et al 1993). Although a health law (1579/85) has been enacted to make provision for, and regulate, the management of medical technology in the public sector (as well as deal with the research and evaluation of technological developments) the appropriate procedures for implementation have not been set up. Furthermore, no such legislative coverage applies to the private sector, with the exception of the arrangements concerning protection against ionic radiation. The mechanisms provided for in the public sector include:

• The setting up of a general directorate of biomedical technology in the Ministry of Health;
• Regulations for the application of such technology in health care;
• Rational use of equipment and technical support;
• Support for production and technological development programmes, and
• Provision of training programmes for health care professionals.

These arrangements were never implemented and are clearly intended to apply primarily to the public sector. At the same time basic problems in health care technologies such as evaluation of medical efficacy, efficiency and rational geographical distribution on the basis of needs and/or population do not exist. Table 5 indicates the unequal geographical distribution of medical technology.

In practice, the accuracy, reliability, effectiveness and efficiency of high level medical technology both in the public and private sector is evaluated on the basis of general information originating from international literature and the information provided by the technology suppliers. The introduction and installation of medical technology in the public sector is based on an empirical and crude rate of needs or on the demand and power of hospital consultants who use mass media to stimulate public interest and pressurise the government to yield to their demands. At the same time, in the private sector, the introduction of high technology depends primarily on the income of the region and the number of doctors. There are no studies in Greece in the field of economic evaluation of medical technology. Furthermore, regulations that could be applied to management in the public sector do not exist, and the prices of products rely more on perceived benefits than on empirical evidence. On the other hand, in the private sector medical technology may be freely installed by commercial

Table 5. Regional allocation of biomedical technology in Greece (per million/inhabitants)

Region	CT Scanners	NMRs	Heart Transplant Centres	Liver Transplant Centres	Kidney Transplant Centres
Athens	12.0	1.6	0.5	0.25	1.0
Thessaloiki	16.0	2.0	1.0	-	1.0
Peloponnesos	5.0	1.0	-	-	-
Thessaly	5.0	-	-	-	-
Central Greece	2.0	-	-	-	-
Crete	4.0	-	-	-	-
Epirus	3.0	-	-	-	-
East Macedonia and Thrace	3.0	-	-	-	-
Ionian Islands	5.0	-	-	-	-
Agean Islands	2.5	-	-	-	-

Source: Department of Health Economics, Athens School of Public Health

and profit-making enterprises and health centres on the conditions laid down by the Ministry of Commerce.

The extensive diffusion of imaging diagnostic medical technology in the private sector in the last three years could be explained by the absence of planning and governmental regulations, and also of effective criteria for financing such services. Financing of the services provided by the centres of medical technology is based on retrospective remuneration for each item out of budgets of the Sickness Funds. This tends to favour demand stimulated by suppliers, since neither any control on them exists nor are the patients charged for care. It has been estimated that in 1991, Sickness Funds spent in the private sector on imaging technology alone 20 billion drachmas (80 million ECU). This development has created a new balance between the public and private sectors. There are clear signs that the former is becoming technologically dependent on the latter especially since 1990, and the priorities of national health policy are changing radically. This dependence is accompanied by significant cuts in the health care public budget, which when combined with increases in the price of the hospital market, is expected to create large deficits in the Sickness Funds budgets.

THE URGENT NEED FOR CHANGE

As it has been pointed out the rapid diffusion of new technology is not necessarily a negative development. Indeed, technology may improve the quality of care and/or reduce costs (Drummond 1987). The question which then arises is: is this true in the Greek case? Are there appropriate mechanisms in operation for encouraging a rational diffusion and use of health technology in Greece? Unfortunately, the answer is no. It is worth noting that the huge expansion of the private sector in high imaging technology in Greece in the last few years in conjunction with the illegal economic transactions between patients and physicians[2] raised important questions on the medical ethics of physicians in Parliament (Committee of Parliament, 1992).

The above problems faced by Greece in the development of health care technology require measures for urgent action. According to Haan and Rutten (1987) two kinds of regulation are possible. Governmental regulations by directive, or, by incentive, or, a combination of both. Given that the Greek health care system is a private-public mix, it is necessary that any measure adapted is not just for the market forces but also for the needs of the population at large. Apart from the need for the introduction of economic evaluation for health technology, a mechanism which demands some time, measures in the financing of such services and restrictions on physicians may have direct effects. More specifically, in the framework of planning one can put forward the following proposals:

- Health technologies such as transplantation centres, C-T scanners and NMRs need to be planned at national level on the basis of a health charter. This charter

---

[2] Studies in health care estimate that the size of the hidden economy in Greece is about 20 per cent of the total health spending (Pavlopoulos 1987; Niakas et al 1990).

would identify the limits on supply in each health region and introduce 'necessity certificates' as part of the process of approval for the installation of special departments and technologies. The certificates would involve an investigation of the medical and economic effectiveness, technological safety, reliability, precision of the proposed technology, and an report of the extent to which it would met the needs of the population.

- Financing methods, the method of reimbursement, and prices of such services must be scrutinized. For example, since the public Sickness Funds are the only buyers on behalf of the insured, such services (patients can not afford to pay out of pocket high costs of medical technology) must be negotiated both for prices and volume. Contracts and payments in a prospective annual basis seem to be appropriate as the literature points out. Another measure is the exclusion of non appropriate technologies from public financing and or in some cases the imposition of high charges to the patient.
- Physician power must be restricted in prescribing high technology services. Because medical audit and peer review are difficult to be implement in Greece at the moment, a measure which does not cover the patient or impose charges on him for C-T and NMR scanners when a doctor at primary level demands such services may be proved very effective.
- Management in public hospitals in which high technology is available must be intensified. Especially, transplantation centres in the public sector must be financed by a central budget and economic, educational and moral incentives must be given to the professionals in such centres. At the same time, economic evaluation must be introduced and comparisons between centres both in the public and private sector will make the agencies and the public to know what it is worth.

CONCLUSIONS

There is no doubt that health care services in Greece which have recently experienced two sets of reforms in diametrically opposed directions, are faced with a series of complex problems both in the financing and provision side. The recent rapid growth of medical technology which overcame even the richer countries in the European Community may add new side effects to the budgets of the Sickness Funds. The large deficits of the latter, and the drastic reduction of family budgets, demand an effective managerial process in health technology. This must include access to appropriate medical technology, cost containment, and no charges to the patient. The present paper suggests a move in this direction towards a dialogue which should provide an insight in formulating a national health policy in biomedical health technology.

REFERENCES

Committee of Parliament (1992): Proceedings on Health Care Issues, Athens.

Drummond MF (1987): Economic Evaluation and the Rational Diffusion and Use of Health Technology, Health Policy, 7, 309-324

Figueras J., Normand Ch., Roberts J., Mckee M., Hunter D., Karokis A., Pope C., Azene G. (1992): Health Care Infrastructure Needs in the Lagging Regions. London School of Hygiene and Tropical Medicine.

Haan GHMG and Rutten FFH(1987): Economic Appraisal, Health Services Planning and Budgetary Management for Health Technologies in Drummond MF(ed). Economic Appraisal of Health Technology in the European Community. Oxford University Press.

KEPE (1988): Five Year Plan for Health. Centre for Planning and Development. Athens

Kyriopoulos J. (1993): Health Expenditures in Greece. Centre for Health Social Sciences. Athens.

Kyriopoulos J., Drizi B., Ktenas E., Kontogeorgaki E., Georgoussi E. (1992): Health Investments in Greece 1970-2000, Health Review, 3, 6(19) 47-51

Kyriopoulos J., Georgoussi E., Ktenas E., Drizi B., Kontogeorgaki E. (1993): Health Expenditures in Greece, 1970-2000, Health Review, 4(1) 20

Niakas D. (1991): Current Cost-Containment Policies in Health Care at International level and the Greek Case, Health Review 2, 3: 27-33

Niakas D. (1992): The New Proposals for Health Care The Quadrature of the Circle? Society, Economy and Health, 1, 1: 3-16

Niakas D., Kyriopoulos J. (1992a): Health Care Resource Allocation in Greece before and after the NHS Establishment: The Case of Public Spending. Paper presented at 4th European Health Services Research Meeting, Paris 16-18 December.

Niakas D., Kyriopoulos J. (1992b): Financing Health Care in Greece and Health Expenditures in: Chytil M. K., Duru G., Eimeren W., Flagle Ch.: Health Systems-the Challenge of Change. Omnipress, Prague.

Niakas D., Skoutelis G. and Kyriopoulos J(1990): Searching the Underground Activity in Health Care Sector: A first approach Review, 6, 42-45

Pavlopoulos P(1987): The Underground Economy in Greece: A Quantitative Determination, IOBE, Athens

7 Training Health Managers for Developing Countries in Developed Countries — Fish Out of Water?

ZILLYHAM ROJAS, PETER SANDIFORD & JAVIER MARTINEZ
Liverpool School of Tropical Medicine

INTRODUCTION

The current trend towards health sector decentralization and the establishment of District Health Systems in many developing countries has highlighted the need for better mid-level management practice (WHO 1990: 3). Many Ministries of Health have devoted considerable resources to ensure management training for their staff, with particular emphasis to those teams or individuals responsible for managing District Health Systems. The result has been a sharp increase in the demand for training and, in consequence, a mushrooming of courses and training programmes in developed countries to meet the demand. Emphasis on training has subsequently reflected in health sector aid budgets: provision of training constitutes an increasingly significant part of official development aid. This paper argues that training, as a form of development assistance is not always an effective way to transfer managerial skills, and that it may provide greater rewards to developed country institutions of higher education than it does to the developing countries themselves for whom the aid was ostensibly intended. The case is made for a shift in focus: where possible training for health managers should be provided in their own country, with the collaboration of in-country training institutions, in the language normally used by the trainees and as close as possible to their working environment.

THE MARKET FOR SHORT COURSES

The emphasis of most past efforts in health management training in developing countries had typically been on conventional training of technical managers from hospitals and central ministries. Training for middle level health managers was largely neglected until the policies of decentralisation led to the proliferation of short courses for middle level health staff in the developed world, particularly within

Strategic Issues in Health Care Management. Edited by M. Malek, J. Rasquinha and P. Vacani
© 1993 John Wiley & Sons Ltd

universities and schools of public health as a way to `help' developing countries to face their challenges.

In the United Kingdom the establishment of new courses for mid-level staff from Developing Countries (LDCs) was also encouraged by the changes to the tuition fee regulations. In 1980 the United Kingdom introduced a policy of charging overseas students full-cost tuition fees. In competing for this lucrative source of income academic institutions have 'repackaged' their offerings and often reduced their standards for admission making their entry requirements more flexible. Williams (1984: 272) argues that "in some instances 'more flexible' means 'lower' or 'easier' and that at some universities and colleges entry standards for students from abroad have dropped". Prospectuses and course brochures are multiplying, and advertisements for courses of study in Britain appear in various foreign newspapers. British higher education institutions now find themselves in a market where the customer calls the tune and where they no longer enjoy the luxury of waiting for students to queue up at their gates with applications (Williams 1984).

However, mushrooming of courses and increased training budgets attached to official development aid have not increased significantly the options that Developing Countries have to train their mid-level managers. Firstly, because more often than not training abroad has been the only choice offered by donors as against, say, in-country training through institutional strengthening. Second, because donors have naturally favoured donor country institutions as training providers, to the extent of excluding any other alternative sources of training. In 1988, for instance, British government supported students who received training in the UK represented 94.7 percent of the total. Only 0.5 percent received training in their own country (Hulme 1990: 22). Donors have often been criticised for providing training to meet "donor needs" such as commercial or political interests, gaining a favourable image in host countries and winning influential friends, rather than considering what might be best for the recipient country (Hulme 1990). Iredale, in his review of training as a component of British ODA assistance concedes that a number of perceptions of its purposes, uses and styles interact at the time of deciding what training might be best for a particular situation. Perceptions range from "the trainee's to those of his/her employer, the ODA's project managers and desk officers, and the institution where the training takes place"(Iredale 1990: iv) Whatever the perceptions "the present fee structure in UK institutions tends to favour the provision of substantial amounts of UK training rather than in-country training which brings in only relatively small consultancy fees and involves sometimes lengthy staff absences". (Iredale 1992: 6)

On the other hand, overseas training also serves the personal interests of individuals and institutions in developing countries at the expense of gains in managerial skills. Ministries of health and recipients of scholarships may regard a scholarship to study abroad as a reward, a vacation, or a "junket" rather than a learning experience (Fry 1984). This can compromise the quality and performance of training participants and affect the attitudes of those who would otherwise be more concerned about their learning responsibilities since just the attendance of an overseas course increases an individual's prestige within an organization. The reward, therefore could be double for some, but quite positive for those with motivation to make changes to improve health. Moreover, it is widely known that some people with influence attend overseas courses attracted for the per diem, as well as some government ministries using scholarships as a way of removing someone from their post, either for political reasons or because of incompetence. Iredale (1992: 2) pointed out that "overseas training will often be a part of a process of patronage, reward, or even getting rid of unwanted staff".

CURRENT APPROACHES AND STRATEGIES FOR TRAINING LDC'S HEALTH MANAGERS

Kerrigan and Luke describe four training approaches for enhancing managerial skills in LDC's (Kerrigan and Luke 1987). They are:

Formal training

This is the conventional type of training and the most common approach encountered. It's emphasis is predominantly on training individuals in classroom settings. Despite efforts by institutions of higher education to broaden the range of teaching methods used, formal training still relies heavily on didactic lecturing.

Formal training is generally provided in a classroom settings with at least one 'teacher' and at least one 'student'. It consists of discrete, time-bound teaching sessions, their contents being presented predominantly as fixed, knowledge modules. It is "usually designed to transmit knowledge, information and techniques efficiently through a variety of methods, and most often presupposes a model of the ideal or desired managerial behaviour" (Kerrigan and Luke 1987: 40).

On-the-job Training

This is the major managerial training approach used by industry in Japan, China, and the United States. It is perhaps also the oldest approach. "The training of senior officials in government historically has been the process of tutelage, in which the style, knowledge, techniques, wisdom, and even ethics of experienced government officials were transmitted personally to their successors" (Kerrigan and Luke 1987: 81). This method ranges from informal and even unintentional learning such as that which occurs whenever a junior manager works with a senior manager to the more formal programme of indoctrination used to prepare administrators for higher posts in an organization. In medicine, it is widely used to train nurses, specialist physicians and surgeons. In primary health care programmes in developing countries on-the-job training is usually considered to be an integral component of supervision. However, this opportunity is not usually fully exploited. This approach is also used in the health sector whenever consultants from overseas work with identified counterparts.

Action Training

Action training (AT) is basically a combination of formal training sessions with on-the-job problem solving. It is a recently developed approach since it has become recognized by the mid-1970's. According to Kerrigan and Luke (1987) AT approach has developed in various forms under variety of names. Perhaps the best known form of AT is under the Action Learning (AL) name which was developed by Reg Revans. Revans is its best known advocate and has published extensively on the techniques and their applications (see Revans 1966; 1980; 1983). The Learning Equation presented by Revans (1987) shows how AL takes into account two starting-points in the process of learning: being told by others and finding out for ourselves. The first is called Programmed instruction (P), and the second is Questioning insight (Q). Learning is denoted by L, therefore the learning equation L = P + Q represents the combination of P, which is in general the learning provided by traditional education and learning, and Q, which is largely the product of action learning. Nevertheless, basically AT in general, involves training the participants in decision-making and action by getting them to solve real-life problems, rather than allowing them to be passive recipients of someone else's wisdom and knowledge. The training includes working in real-life situations in a particular project or programme and is related to specific here-and-now problems. An important characteristic of AT is that it not only emphasizes individual skills building, but also the evolution of team skills and general organizational development. When AT is applied, the majority of time is given to identify the problems, and to applying any training solutions to the problems that may be suggested. The application of this approach in the health sector is reported by Revans (1980) in his form of AL, and claimed that it strengthened management in some of the British National Health Service (NHS) hospitals. Clutterbuck and Crainer (1991) described the improvements achieved by Revans in 10 NHS hospitals as exceptional, since he proved that health staff were able to identify their problems and find ways to solve them by working and learning from each other in real-life situations. Cassels and Janovsky (1991) have described a similar process for strengthening the management capacity of district and provincial health management teams clearly based on principles of AT, although they do not claim to applied have AT.

Non-Formal Training

This is essentially self-directed learning through peers. It can be described as a learning situation where a group of peers share expertise, exchange practical ideas, and inform each other of emerging trends, issues, or theories. Although it is typically neglected as a viable management training approach for developing countries, it does occur spontaneously in a variety of organizational forms from highly structured clubs to loosely structured networks or support groups.

Of the four training approaches, formal training is the one most often provided by institutions in Europe and the United States in spite of the fact that this approach is not the one with the greatest potential to achieve the immediate management training objectives. Figure 1 summarises the analysis of the relative advantages of each approach (Kerrigan and Luke 1987). Of the four, AT would appear to offer the most, perhaps because it combines the benefits of formal training with those of on-the-job training.

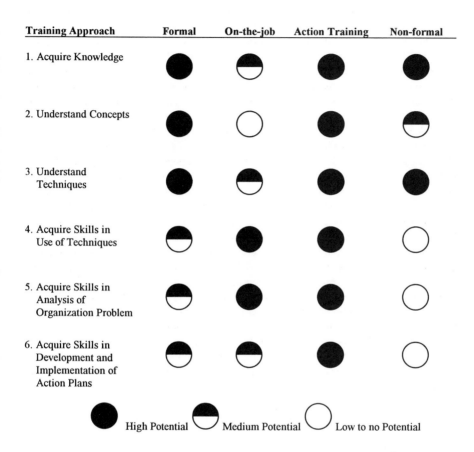

Figure 1. Inherent potential for achieving Selective Immediate objects[1]

THE PROBLEMS OF TRAINING HEALTH MANAGERS IN DEVELOPED COUNTRIES

The Problem of Language and Context

Study abroad provides one of the most effective means to acquire skills in a foreign language (Fry 1984). However important competency in a foreign language might be it is not particularly important for professionals working in the periphery where district health managers work. When taking a short training course abroad in a

---

[1] Kerrigan and Luke (1987: 161) presented this figure including a long-term objective. Similar results as in this figure were observed.

language different from the one they would normally use at work, communication may become a major constraint.

While it will remain valuable to provide high quality training within universities to train health management trainees or large hospitals managers from developing countries in developed countries, it is unquestionable that training for district health managers will be most effective if it recognises the needs, conditions, and health sector organization of each country and its culture. This is not possible with third country training if participants come from markedly different backgrounds. Kerrigan and Luke (1987) point out that not only are managerial skills in developing countries different from those regarded as effective in industrialized countries, but also they differ from country to country. Hence, the wholesale transfer of theories, concepts and tools from developed countries to developing countries should be avoided. Whatever knowledge is transmitted, it must be adapted to the specific culture of the learner to lower the other major difficulty in translating classroom learning to behavioural changes on the job. "The closer the job training occurs the greater the likelihood of relevance the training can best be done" (Baum and Tolbert 1985: 133)

Moreover, it is very difficult for a course designer to find subjects and recreate scenarios matching the specific needs of health managers working in intermediate levels such as District, particularly when trainees come from different countries and backgrounds, have different individual abilities for learning, are used to different learning styles and interpret certain situations differently. To prevent the class-room becoming a Tower of Babel, teaching has to be made sufficiently general to be relevant or comprehensible to most of the participants, the result of this is that much of the significance, relevance and therefore learning opportunities from the materials presented are lost. A course may merely result in learning other ways of seeing things generally.

The Problem of Approaches

There is probably no single best training approach for health managers from developing countries, let alone for management in general. Kerrigan and Luke (1987) conclude that training needs are most likely to be met if an eclectic combination of the four main approaches is used; experimenting with different combinations of training approaches will be needed prior to deciding on the best mix. However, a major problem of training health managers from developing countries in developed countries is that one is very much restricted to the use of formal training in a classroom environment. When referring to health management courses provided in the United Kingdom, Riseborough and Walter (1988: 108) conclude that "what is required to complement the formal (academic) management course is an approach which seeks to identify the changes and developments required, and the unresolved problems encountered, at a specific time within an organization".

There are several reasons why other approaches are not used and which bias educational institutions towards formal training. Firstly, courses based in developed countries are unable to use real-life situations, or managerial problems from health institutions that would be relevant in developing countries. Even those new efforts to develop practical exercises, role plays and simulations are frequently criticized for being unrealistic and not relevant for most students in their actual jobs. Also, they must inevitably lack the element of 'risk' which plays such a fundamental role in management decisions. For example, it becomes relatively easy to decide on staff transfers or cuts in drugs budgets when these decisions are taken in a class-room situation: in this context whether the scenario recreated is fictional or real remains unimportant. Only Real-life situations can bring this out since health management development "is more likely to be successful if the focus is on problems of real and immediate concern of the managers involved...". In addition, "Different actors will see problems in their own way and, following from this, the way problems are defined often points to a particular kind of solution" (WHO 1990: 18-19).

Secondly, the historically narrow conception of training, characterized by teaching knowledge in a classroom setting that emphasizes dependency on experts. There is a need to make a conceptual distinction between `learning' and `teaching'. Formal courses will tend to predominate as long as training is viewed in terms of teaching or instruction offered in a classroom setting. Rather, training should be viewed as providing learning opportunities and not simply as teaching. Learning results in a relatively permanent change in behaviour or perspective that occurs as a result of practice, experience, or reflection.

Thirdly, most trainers are continuously developing their own techniques and methods as they gain experience, and there is more likely that they have a 'pet' method, or they merely reproduce the methods in which they themselves were trained, or which is traditional in the institution where they work (Kerrigan and Luke, 1987). In addition other factors like costs to produce and acquire experience in a developing country could be a constraint, as well as the size of a training group that can be an important factor in using a particular approach.

Finally, the prestige of overseas universities, and the patterns of incentives and rewards stressing the possession of an academic education credential or certificate are very attractive for any person from developing country. This situation creates the demand for training under the formal approach. On the other hand, donors funding patterns and aid packages have kept supporting the demand, since there is not enough evidence of the effectiveness of other approaches due to difficulties of evaluation. However, the ODA, World Bank and WHO have already recognized the appropriateness of using in-country and in-service training approaches (Iredale 1992; Baum and Tolbert 1985; WHO 1990).

The Problem of Cost

Strategically, the high costs of training in Europe and North America mean that even if such training were effective, the number of students who could benefit from it will only be a small minority of the developing world's middle level health managers. While in-country training has several potential advantages because the wide flexibility to use all four training approaches to enhance the managerial talent of its health staff, its major disadvantage is that high-quality trainers may be scarce, which forces the use of less effective indigenous trainers. The problem of shortage of trainers is exacerbated by the limited language skills of many of the management trainers from developed countries who seldom speak the language used by trainees at work. On the other hand, the establishment of training programmes in large countries or for regional groups of countries with similar health systems can help to get around the problem of the shortage of skilled trainers.

The Problem of Institutional Strengthening

Developed country training does a lot to strengthen academic and teaching institutions in the developed world, but does so at the expense of similar institutions in the developing world which struggle to gain experience in this field. According to Iredale (1992: 5) "in allocating a group of foreign students to a UK institution for training we are in effect providing support in an indirect way to the UK institution", he added that this practice of bringing people to train "could be read as a tacit acknowledgement of the inadequacy of their owns country's training capability". The key solution seems to be in establishing links between the academic institutions of the developed and developing countries and support the developing country's institution in upgrading and strengthening the capacity of its academic institutions.

Nevertheless, the need for basing training programmes with international expertise in developing countries is now being recognised, and a number of in-country courses has been established under various headings of health management and public health.

The Problem of the Lack of Evidence about the Effectiveness of Training Provided

Hulme (1990) when addressing the issue of the effectiveness of British aid for training, recognises that regardless of the success or failure of the training aid, most donors, recipients and providers have favourable comments on the results obtained. However, methodologies for evaluation of training remain subjective and not systematic. Most of the evaluation exercises occurs at a level far from the actual impact on the output of the trainees in their organization. Evaluation exercises

> commence with evaluation of the quality of the training input itself; next is the trainee's reaction to a training activity and opinions on its potential use; then come evaluations of the proximate impact of training on the individual (in terms of learning and performance). (Hulme 1990: 13)

He adds that evaluators, rightly or wrongly, use these exercises to make inferences about the results achieved at the other level such as the impact of the output. As a result, most of evaluation materials focus on 'improving' training aid practice rather than 'proving' its contribution to enhance the trainee's average job performance. Tziner and Haccoun (1991: 167) pointed out that "the ultimate purpose of training evaluation must be to assess the level of on-the-job training transfer".

Nevertheless, evaluation of the effects of health management training courses for developing countries is extremely difficult. There is "little actual experience of assessing whether expected improvements in the performance of health and management systems are taking place" (WHO 1990: 1).

SIGLOS — AN ALTERNATIVE HEALTH MANAGEMENT TRAINING

Despite some evidence that management training is having rather less impact than one might have hoped, there have been few attempts to date to solve the problems that have been identified. The SIGLOS Project, a training programme in information systems for district health managers from spanish-speaking Central America is, nevertheless, one such attempt. SIGLOS tries to meet not only existing learning needs and develop indigenous capacity, but also includes a significant follow-up component to evaluate the extent to which the skills acquired by the participants are later applied in their daily practice.

The core of the programme is a six week intensive course to be held annually in Costa Rica. It will employ a mixture of various formal training methods and action learning, based in four nearby district health systems. The medical director of each one will identify a management problem or issue which s/he would like tackled by the course participants who will be divided into groups for this purpose. Each group will have a tutor to provide guidance in how to gather the necessary information, analyse it, and present it to district health managers and other relevant decision-makers.

The project's other component consists of a number of case studies to be carried out by course graduates upon return to their workplace. The purpose of these is to demonstrate whether or not the skills acquired during the course can be put into practice, and to identify factors which may be limiting the impact on the management of health care delivery. Lessons drawn from these case studies will be used to modify the content or training methods in subsequent years of the course.

The SIGLOS project was developed jointly by the Liverpool School of Tropical Medicine and the Costa Rican Institute of Research and Training in Nutrition and Health (INCIENSA), with seeding funds from the Overseas Development Administration. The level of UK financial and technical support for the course will diminish each year in the expectation that the training programme will become self-sustaining within three years.

It might be asked why health information systems for local management was selected as the focus of the training rather than simply management. There are several reasons, but above all, it was felt very strongly that managers fail not because of inability to make decisions (although this can also be a problem), but because they fail to make *informed* decisions. Information systems (in the broadest sense of the term) are needed to improve the quality of decision-making in areas related to the planning and monitoring of health service provision. The result should be improved managerial decisions leading to improved health system efficiency and effectiveness (Sandiford, Annett, and Cibulskis 1992).

Furthermore, the attempts by all countries in Central America to develop District Health Systems (Sistemas Locales de Salud or SILOS), where some devolution of decision-making is implicit, have made it apparent that information systems need to be reoriented to fit the requirements of district level decision-makers. There is now a pressing shortage of managers with the skills to identify their data needs and determine the most appropriate means of collection and analysis, but also able to transform data into information conducive to improve health service delivery. As Central America is a region with rapidly increasing numbers of microcomputers in the public sector, the ability to make effective use of a information technology has become imperative.

The need for training in health information systems has been recognised by Central American governments themselves, and was a recurring theme in their submission to the Third Madrid Conference for "Health and Peace for Development and Democracy" (PAHO 1991). It was also highlighted in a recent study of the health sector in Central America (Sandiford and Rojas 1992).

HOW DOES SIGLOS AVOID THE SHORTCOMINGS OF TRADITIONAL, DEVELOPED COUNTRY, HEALTH MANAGEMENT TRAINING?

The SIGLOS project has been designed specifically to avoid the main pitfalls of previous approaches to strengthening the health management skills of developing countries. There are several features of the SIGLOS project which serve this aim.

The Language and Context

SIGLOS will be located in a leading Central American health research and training institution (INCIENSA) and will be taught in the local language. This will ensure that the course focuses on the operational realities of health systems in Central America.

Though the general health status in Costa Rica -where SIGLOS will be located- differs markedly from that in Guatemala, Honduras, El Salvador, Nicaragua and Panamá, health systems in these sister countries are very similar and to some extent converging. This should enhance participants to apply their newly acquired skills in the specific circumstances encountered in their own countries. In other words, the fish will remain in water.

The Approach

Since the course will take place in a developing country, the action training approach can and will be used. District Health Systems of Costa Rica will collaborate with SIGLOS in providing real-life issues and problems which require evaluation or investigation. Course participants will work within Costa Rican District Health

Systems in data collection and analysis, to then present alternatives for action to District Health Managers.

The major characteristics of action learning as described by Martineau (1992) can be incorporated within the SIGLOS project. These are:

- **More 'questioning insight' (Q) than 'programmed learning' (P) in the 'learning' (L) equation L = P + Q.** The SIGLOS course will have less sessions of formal training (P) than action learning (Q) by tackling real-life problems within the workplace.
- **A cycle of action and reflection:** Since training is related to here-and-now problems, action itself becomes the centre for training. To complete the cycle, there will be reflection sessions which discuss and analyse the achievements, and any obstacles encountered.
- **Action based on dealing with significant problems:** Health management problems will be identified according to specific needs of real actors, and situations.
- **Fellows working together in sets:** The course will be organized in work teams, and each team will have to deal with a specific problem of a District Health System.
- **Most of the learning coming within the set:** Each team will probably require a fair amount of guidance from tutors to get the process going but, once under way, learning will occur as team members tackle problems by themselves.

Costs

In Central America, where the nations are small, it is difficult to justify developing separate training programmes for each country. A more rational strategy is to support regionally based training in institutions of proven worth. A training programme which serves a single small country will often become unsustainable once the immediate needs of that country are met since the numbers required to replace losses though natural attrition are insufficient to guarantee the course's viability. Regionally based training permits the concentration of expertise and spreads the cost of capital items such as the microcomputer laboratory which will be almost impossible to provide in each country.

The advantages of regional strategy are particularly acute in Central America, where there have been serious efforts to co-ordinate policies, programmes and activities in the health sector (Sandiford and Rojas 1992).

It is intended that SIGLOS will become self-sustaining and run virtually entirely by staff of Central America within a period of three years. Although initially there will be substantial input from British trainers, this assistance will diminish steadily as SIGLOS becomes established, and acquires prestige and recognition by Ministries of Health and key NGO's. The course will eventually become self-financed from tuition fees paid by Ministries and NGO's who will sponsor participants in the same way as they sponsor participants on more expensive courses in developed countries. As the course will be held in Central America with predominantly Central American trainers, costs can be kept well below those of equivalent courses in Europe or North America.

Institutional Strengthening

In contrast to the courses run in European or North American training institutions, SIGLOS will become a product of a Latin American training institution. The institution (INCIENSA) will be strengthened by the investment in a microcomputer laboratory, but more importantly, by the contact with experts from both Europe and Latin America on different areas related to health management and health information systems who will participate in the training programme. The knowledge and experience of European and Latin American experts is expected to safeguard the quality of the learning process, and will ensure that contemporary thought in the field of health management and information systems is not neglected. The prestige of a developed country university training is transferred to the developing country institution by the involvement of developed country university trainers.

CONCLUSIONS

It is too soon to know whether this project can succeed where developed country management training has failed, but one of the main concerns of the project is to ensure that the skills imparted are put into practice when participants return to their normal working environment. Follow-up and evaluation is therefore an important component and will be based upon the management changes brought about in the aforementioned case studies.

Should the project prove successful the case for developed country based training for mid-level managers provided at increasingly high costs could hardly be justified. Fish would the remain in water. After all, should not tropical fish swim in tropical waters?

REFERENCES

America and Mexico, Commissioned by the Overseas Development Administration, Liverpool Associates in Tropical Health, Liverpool.

Baum, W. Ch. and Tolbert, S.M. (1985), Investing in Development: Lessons of World Bank Experience, Oxford University Press, New York.

Burgoyne, J. and Stuart, R. (1978), Management Development: Context and Strategies, Gower Press, England.

Cassels, A. and Janovsky, K. (1991), Strengthening Health Management in Districts and Provinces Handbook for Facilitators, WHO/SHS/DHS/91.3, World Health Organization, Geneva.

Clutterbuck, D. and Crainer, S. (1991), Los Maestros del Management: Hombres que Llegaron más Lejos, Grijalbo, Barcelona.

Eskin, F. (1986), 'Measuring the Effect of Training Courses on the Participants', Journal of Management in Medicine, 1 (1), 58-67.

Fry, G. W. (1984), 'The Economic and Political Impact of Study Abroad', Comparative Education Reviews, 28 (2), 203-220.

Hall, D. and Cockburn, E. (1990), 'Developing Management Skills', Management Education and Development, 21 (1), 41-50.

Huczynski, A. (1983), Encyclopedia of Management Development Methods, Gower, England.

Hulme, D. (1990), The Effectiveness of British Aid for Training, Action Aid Development Report, London.

Iredale, R. (1992), The Power of Change, Part 1: A Review of Training: Needs and Criteria, Overseas Development Administration, London.

Kerrigan, J.E. and Luke, J.S. (1987), Management Training Strategies for Developing Countries, Lynne Rienner Publishers, Colorado.

Martineau, T. (1992), Action Learning and the Marlboro Country: Lessons for Health Management Development, Liverpool School of Tropical Medicine, Liverpool, (Unpublished document).

PAHO (1991), Third Madrid Conference: Health and Peace for Development and Democracy, Central American Health Initiative, PPSCAP 1991-1995, Second Phase, May 1991, PAHO/WHO, Washington.

Revans, R. W. (1987), 'International Perspectives on Action Learning', Manchester Training Handbook No 9, Institute of Development Policy and Management, University of Manchester.

Revans, R. W. (1983), The ABC of Action Learning Chartwell-Bratt, Kent.

Revans, R. W. (1980), Action Learning Blond and Briggs, London.

Revans, R. W. (1966), The Theory of Practice in Management, Macdonald, London.

Riseborough, P.A. and Walter, A. (1988), Management in Health Care, Wrigh, London.

Sandiford, P. and Rojas, Z. (1992), A Desk Study of the Health Sector in Central

Sandiford, P. Annett, H. and Cibulskis, R. (1992), 'What Can Information Systems do for Primary Health Care', Social Science and Medicine, 34 (10), 1077-1087.

Systems for Primary Health Care, WHO/SHS/DH/88.1/Rev 1, Geneva.

Tziner, A. and Haccoun, R. (1991), 'Personal and Situational Characteristics influencing the Effectiveness of Transfer of Training Improvement Strategies', Journal of Occupational Psychology, 64, 167-177.

Williams, P. (1984), 'Britain's Full-Cost Policy for Overseas Students', Comparative Education Reviews, 28 (2), 258-278.

World Health Organization (1990), Management Development for Primary Health Care: Report of a Consultation, 28 May-1 June 1990, Geneva.

World Health Organization (1988), The Challenge of Implementation: District Health

8 Innovative Strategies to Improve Clinic Planning & Management — The Case of a Paediatric Clinic in Iowa

MARIANN E. KRALL, JEANNE M. GOCHE & CLAIBOURNE I. DUNGY

University of Iowa Hospitals and Clinics, USA

INTRODUCTION

As the delivery of health care shifts from the in-patient to the ambulatory setting, there is increasing pressure to improve the quality of care and the effectiveness of health care delivery in the outpatient arena. Unfortunately, administrators, physicians, and staff are provided with few models to serve as benchmarks to evaluate ambulatory clinic performance. This is particularly true for academic centres that have the added responsibility of providing an environment that is conducive for teaching and research, whilst at the same time maximizing the efficiency and effectiveness of health care service delivery. Faced with these challenges, the University of Iowa Hospitals and Clinics (UIHC) elected to adopt selected strategies from Total Quality Management (TQM) theory and computer simulation to assess proposed changes in the delivery of ambulatory health care services.

The University of Iowa Hospitals and Clinics is a large academic medical centre which has approximately 460,000 clinic visits annually and is located in Iowa City, Iowa (population 60,000). The mission of the UIHC is three-fold: patient care, teaching, and research. The UIHC provides in-patient and out-patient services covering 125 medical specialties. This paper focuses on the improvement process which was implemented and supported by clinic staff in the multi-specialty Paediatric Outpatient Clinic.

GETTING STARTED

In 1989, the UIHC began implementation of TQM on an institution-wide basis. This involved a quality improvement process incorporating the approaches of Deming

Strategic Issues in Health Care Management. Edited by M. Malek, J. Rasquinha and P. Vacani
© 1993 John Wiley & Sons Ltd

(Deming, 1987), Juran (Juran, 1988, 1989), and others. The quality improvement process outlined in table 1 serves as a guide to address project organization, problem diagnosis, solution development, and continuous monitoring for future improvements. This guide also lists quality improvement techniques appropriate for the various steps in the process.

The Paediatric Outpatient Clinic was identified as an area of operation which needed focused management attention due to increased demands on the clinic. Approximately 28,000 patient visits were encountered in the Paediatric Out-patient Clinic during 1991-92, a 15% increase in clinic visits over 1987-88. In addition, the Paediatric Cardiology Clinic was to be incorporated into the Paediatric Outpatient Clinic. This merger would add 2,300 visits per year to the Paediatric Outpatient Clinic.

Issues to be evaluated included patient expectations, staff expectations, clinic efficiency, clinic room utilization, patient wait times, provider time with patients, and standard operating procedures. The strategy used to evaluate these issues has three components:

1) creation of a cross functional team
2) application of the UIHC quality improvement process and
3) computerized simulation of clinic flow

IMPLEMENTATION

The first step was selection of the cross-functional team which included administrators, physicians, nurses, and other support staff. The team updated the clinic mission statement and discussed future directions and problems. An important source of information about clinic performance was the 'Examination Room Utilization and Patient Flow Study'. This study was conducted throughout the medical centre in 1991, and provided information regarding clinic room utilization, provider time with patient, patient wait time, and length of clinic visit. The paediatric cross-functional team developed parallel initiatives implementing selected techniques of the quality improvement process.

Bench Marking

The first task was to determine methods and strategies employed by other academic medical centres to address the issues of clinic management, patient volume, and space demands. An exhaustive literature search and discussions with representatives of professional organizations indicated few models existed that were appropriate to assess the complex interactions occurring in an ambulatory clinic setting. Studies from other academic medical centres could not be transferred to the UIHC setting because of differences in study assumptions or methodologies.

A University of Wisconsin Medical Centre examination room utilization rate focused primarily on study methods and did not provide substantive data for comparison (Riley et. al. 1982). When the methods suggested by a 1987 University of Michigan Medical Centre study were employed, the comparison did not produce stable results that could be contrasted with the observed UIHC utilization data (Eady, et. al. 1982). Thus, neither study was able to satisfy UIHC interest in bench marking.

Table 1.　Quality Improvement Process

		QUALITY IMPROVEMENT TECHNIQUES	
(1) PROJECT ORGANIZATION AND DEFINITION			
Goal —Develop a problem statement that describes the problem in specific terms, where it occurs, when it happens, and its extent			
A.	Identify and list problems	Brainstorming Nominal Group Process Pareto	Flow Chart Check Sheet
B.	Determine customers	Brainstorming Input-Process-Output-Model	Flow Chart
C.	Clarify customer expectations and establish quality indicators	Survey Focus Group Brainstorming	Check Sheet
D.	Construct problem statement: identify gap between present and future outcomes	Run chart Histogram Pie Chart Stratification	Pareto Check Sheet Flow Chart
(2) DIAGNOSTIC JOURNEY			
Goal —Develop a complete picture of all of the possible causes of the problem; then agree on the basic causes			
A	Analyze symptoms of the problem	Brainstorming	
B.	Formulate theories of causes	Nominal Group Technique	
C.	Test causes	Scatter Diagram	
D.	Identify root causes	Check Sheet Pareto Cause and Effect Diagram	
(3) REMEDIAL JOURNEY			
Goal —Develop an effective and implementable solution and action plan			
A.	Consider alternative solutions	Brainstorming	
B.	Design solutions and controls	Force Field Analysis	
C.	Address resistance to change	Pie Chart Bar Graphs Flow Chart Solution Selection Matrix	
(4) CONTINUOUS IMPROVEMENT CYCLE			
Goal —Implement the solution and establish needed monitoring procedures and measures			
A.	Implement solutions	Pareto	
B.	Check performance	Histogram	
C.	Monitor control systems	Stratification Control Chart Process Capability	

*Techniques are not all inclusive, nor need all be used in each step.

From: *University of Iowa Hospitals and Clinics Quality Improvement Team Training, Module 1: Introduction to Total Quality Management, University of Iowa Hospitals and Clinics, Iowa City, Iowa, USA 11/91.*

Introspection

The team then performed an internal assessment of clinic operations. Internal assessment requires an openness and willingness to undergo careful self-examination while involving staff from all levels of the organization and, in particular, the staff directly involved with daily operation of the clinic selected for an in-depth evaluation. The team identified several issues that impacted cross functional systems, i.e., administrative units, institutional culture, social systems, and computer applications.

Informal interviews of staff were conducted to gather perceptions of clinic function. The team also compiled a list of problems impeding clinic efficiency. The team carefully examined each item's applicability to the task of improving clinic operations. Selected items underwent further investigation.

Priorities and Quantification

Analysis of data from the Examination Room Utilization and Patent Flow Study was used to determine a priority list of concerns. The boundaries of who and what would be involved and the magnitude of the problem were also assessed. The team used statistical analysis and nominal techniques to identify these characteristics. Sub-specialty clinic volumes and patient profile factors were considered when the Monday morning session was selected for closer review.

Flowcharting

The largest volume Paediatric subspecialty clinics included Allergy/Pulmonary, Cardiology, Child Health (General Paediatrics), Endocrinology, Haematology/Oncology, and Neurology. Flow chart diagrams were created based on input from clinic staff and physicians to document the clinic work and patient flow. A sample flowchart of the Allergy/Pulmonary Clinic is provided in Figure 1. Each sub-specialty clinic flowchart was validated by the appropriate clinic staff and was used in building the simulation models.

SIMULATION STRATEGIES

Identifying the underlying reasons contributing to problems and developing appropriate solutions are among management's greatest challenges. It was noted that intuitive actions did not always yield the desired outcomes. In fact, some past suggestions to increase patient flow and/or efficiency actually created greater problems. These failures served to undermine staff morale and their willingness to be innovative. Hence, finding alternative methods to evaluate changes was a desirable outcome.

Computer simulation of operational processes for health care planning can be used to assist in the evaluation of operational flow and space requirements in

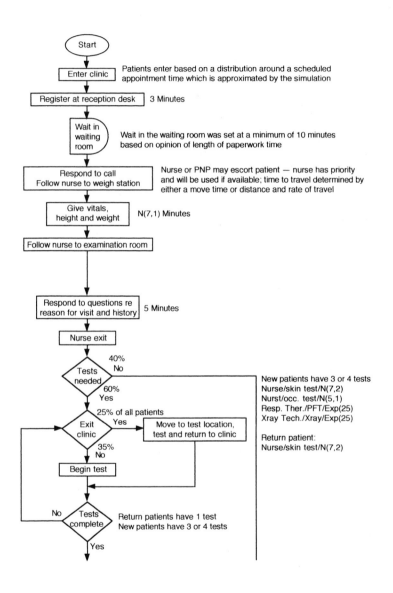

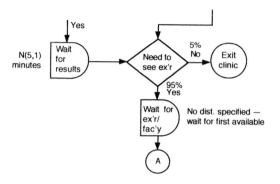

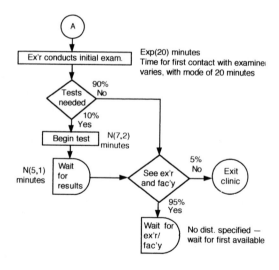

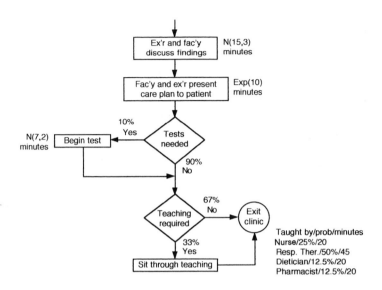

Figure 1.

ambulatory care clinics.   Simulation allows dynamic assessment of operational alternatives without expense or disruption. The construction and evaluation of the simulation model is based on the input of the staff involved in the modelled work process. The techniques and tools used in the planning process provide the basic data and information that can lead to the development of successful simulation models. The decision to use simulation models should be based on the following criteria:

- the systems require high human involvement;
- the work processes are standardized, yet variable; and
- the potential operational changes are expensive and/or disruptive.

Simulation is a dynamic alternative that can be used when there is uncertainty in the system (ProModel Corporation, 1992). The models should be built to represent what is most likely to take place because of the interaction and dependencies between events. Although process exceptions do occur, the exceptions are not likely to cause an entire system to fail. Exceptions should be kept in the proper perspective, and if exceptions are issues, such as in disaster planning, then the exception processes should be simulated separately.

TECHNICAL ASPECTS OF SIMULATION

Simulation models must be constructed with the right emphasis to maximize the likelihood that the results have utility. The three phases for successful model building (preparation, development, and alternatives) and their underlying steps are outlined below.

Preparation

The first step in the process of simulation is to define the purpose of the simulation, which is then used to define decision variables and determine which operational aspects should be modelled. This step is critical to the success of simulation. The decision variables for one of the paediatric sub-specialty clinics included staff utilization rates and patient throughput.

The next step in the preparation process is to define operational locations and/or the fixed physical resources, such as laboratories, stationary equipment, and examination rooms. Patient (entity) and resource (staff and equipment) paths and the number of resources must then be defined. It is important to assess which resources directly contribute to the accuracy of the decision variable(s). Extraneous resources consume computer system resources and unnecessarily complicate the simulation model. Including breakdowns of patient classes can enhance outpatient statistics and the flow of the patient entity within a simulation model. Again, detailed categorizations complicate the model unnecessarily unless they contribute to model validity and accuracy.

The above cautions also apply to the identification of activities and length of time factors that form the processing engine within simulation software. In health care modelling projects, staff may claim that the environment is too unpredictable for modelling. However, situations occurring in a daily clinic are random within bounds. Consequently, activity distributions were generated for the paediatric sub-specialty clinic through analysis of volume information and interviews with clinic staff. Characterization of activities as distributions produces a dynamic and realistic simulation of process interactions. Samples of activities and distributions used for the subspecialty model are given in table 2.

The final preparation step is to determine a timing and frequency for patient arrivals. Similar to the definition of activities, patient arrivals (or inter-arrival times) can be described using distributions in accordance to a prescribed timing. In this model, patients arrived in accordance to the patient schedule with an exponential distribution as shown in table 2. Since patient arrival patterns do not necessarily follow the scheduling pattern, sample values from the 1991 Examination Room Utilization and Patient Flow Study were used to generate appropriate distribution values.

Table 2. Simulation Parameters- Allergy Pulmonary

Resources	Activities	Distribution
Examination Rooms - 5	Create Entities	Exp (13)
Nurse - 1	Register	Constant 3 minutes
Paediatric Nurse Practitioner (PNP) - 2	Paperwork	Constant 10 minutes
Faculty - 1	Vitals	Normal x=7
Examiner (Trainee & Fellow) - 2	History	Constant 5 minutes
Respiratory Therapist (RT) - 2	Test	Exp (25)
Teachers (Pharmacist & Dietician)-2	Wait for Result	Normal x=5 SD=1
X-ray Technician (XT) - 1	Initial Examination	Exp (20)
Clerk - 1	Consult	Normal x=15 SD=3
	Patient Review	Exp (10)
	Nurse Teaches	Constant 20 minutes
	RT Teaches	Constant 45 minutes
	Teachers Teach	Constant 20 minutes
	Schedule	Constant 3 minutes
	Terminate	After 15 Entities or 285 mins

Probabilities

Initial Testing:
35% of patients require one test
25% of patients require three - four tests (50/50 chance)
40% of patients do not require a test

Wait for Results:
95% of patients discuss results
5% of patients leave after initial test(s)

Tests after Review
10% of patients have to have another test
90% of patients continue with examination process

Teaching:
67% of patients do not require teaching
33 % of patients require teaching
Who teaches?
25% require nurse to teach
50% require RT to teach
25% require a pharmacist or dietician to teach

Conditions added later: PNP could serve as nurse or examiner if not busy. Patients arrive in accordance with predetermined-schedule with some variance

Development

The next phase of the process involves the development of a simulation model. The key elements are outlined in Table 3. Clinic staff involvement is critical to the process of model development because of their knowledge of clinic operations, clinic personnel, and the mission of the clinic. In addition, their involvement in meaningful aspects of model development increases the likelihood that they will understand the capability of the simulation model and support its use as an evaluation tool.

Table 3. Preparation steps for simulation modelling

i.	Define Purpose or Objective	- reasons and decision variables
ii.	Define Locations	- physical constraints and where events happen
iii.	Define Path Networks	- travel or movement by resources or entities
iv.	Define Resources	- human and non-human resources and capacities
v.	Define Entities	- distinct types and classes
vi.	Define Processes	- important activities and how long they take
vii.	Define Arrivals	- when and how frequently entities are introduced into the model

The paediatric sub-specialty clinic review included examination of process times, staff utilization and output statistics. In-depth exploration of processes helped to identify unnecessary tasks and ways to improve the flow of the Paediatric Outpatient Clinic. The simulation of one sub-specialty clinic increased awareness of clinic-wide resource interactions and patient flow. The discovery of inefficiencies within the process structure was an important product of the simulation. The simulation also helped to evaluate how effective proposed changes would be in terms of overall staff utilization and patient throughputs. Figure 2 illustrates staff utilization for selected alternatives.

Statistics concerning total length of time in clinic, operation time, wait time, bottlenecks, etc., are generated by simulation software packages for specified patients and clinic staff. The simulation is dynamic due to the representation of activities as distributions and interaction between events. Therefore, the model should be run multiple times to ensure stability and validity over time. Averaging statistics over multiple replications rather than placing too much emphasis on a single output is highly recommended. Methods of evaluating the results from a dynamic simulation model include the calculation of a 'moving average' (Law and Kelton 1991). Tracking the upper bound, lower bound, and mode values are also helpful when trying to interpret change impacts.

Alternative Models

Once the simulation model has been developed and validated, alternatives can be evaluated. The results from alternative models can be used to assess the impact of potential changes on clinic operations and costs. Standard statistical tests should be used to determine the significance of differences between results of various models. If significant differences are substantiated, then more detailed analysis of the alternative models are indicated.

IMPACTS

The UIHC quality improvement process along with state-of-the-art computer simulation facilitated the evaluation of the UIHC Paediatric Outpatient Clinic operation. The process has resulted in substantive changes in the operation of the Paediatric Outpatient Clinic, including clinic staffing patterns, paper flow, and sub-specialty examination room assignments. The process has also triggered the reassessment of trainee education in the clinic and suggestions for improved computer outputs for clinic use have been made. Thus, this process has provided the opportunity to objectively evaluate clinic operations and has resulted in recommendations for improvement which are acceptable to clinic personnel.

CONCLUSION

Administrators, faculty, and staff at the UIHC have developed an innovative strategy to improve the planning and management of ambulatory clinics. This strategy was developed in response to changes in the health care delivery system in the United States. The changes are placing pressure on ambulatory clinics to improve their efficiency and respond to increasing patient volume while experiencing fiscal resource constraints. While all ambulatory clinics must adjust to the changes occurring in the health care delivery system, the response of an academic centre must take into consideration its unique roles of teaching and research when developing strategies to evaluate ambulatory clinics.

The ambulatory clinic patient flow process represents a dynamic and variable environment. The computer simulation model provides a powerful resource for evaluating the clinic environment without the disruption and expense associated with trial and error. The unique nature of the computer simulation is its flexibility. This flexibility allows transfer of the methodology within and between institutions seeking a benchmark to evaluate their performance.

The utility of simulation extends beyond the clinic setting and can be applied to such things as, laboratory services, support services, ancillary services, paperwork, and nursing functions. Virtually any operational process that can be described in a quantitative manner can be evaluated using a dynamic simulation software package. The use of simulation as a planning and assessment tool in health care is not new, but today's powerful simulation products are easier to use and understand for administrators, medical staff, and engineers.

ACKNOWLEDGEMENT

The authors are deeply appreciative to William Petasnick, Chief Operating Officer, The University of Iowa Hospitals and Clinics and Frank H. Morris, Jr., M.D., Head, Department of Paediatrics, The University of Iowa for their encouragement and support. The authors would also like to thank Mrs Pat Moore for preparation of the manuscript.

REFERENCES

Deming, W.E. (1986), *Out of the Crisis*, MIT Press, Cambridge, Massachusetts.

Eady, C., Bame, S., et. al. (1983), 'Characteristics of Outpatient Room Utilization', *Journal of Ambulatory Care Management*, 6, 43-56.

Juran, J.M. (1989), *Juran on Leadership for Quality*, The Free Press, New York.

Juran, J.M. (1988), *Juran on Planning for Quality*, The Free Press, New York.

Law, A.M. and Kelton, D.W. (1991), *Simulation Modelling and Analysis*, 2nd ed., McGraw-Hill Book Company, New York.

Merry, M.D. (1990), 'Total Quality Management for Physicians: Translating the New Paradigm', *Quality Review Bulletin*, 16 (3), 101-105.

ProModel Corporation (1992), *Simulation Modelling for Healthcare Systems: Simulation Training Workshop*, ProModel Corporation, Orem, Utah.

Riley, G.T., Cheung, F.H. and Brower, L.S. (1982), 'Development of an Ambulatory Care Space Utilization Reporting System', *Journal of Ambulatory Care Management*, 5(4), 24-33.

Vogel, L.L. (1989), 'Special Feature: Issues in Patient Care Scheduling at a Large Teaching Hospital', *Journal of Ambulatory Care Management*, 12 (4), 61-69.

Waters, S. (1991), *Computer Simulation: Preventive Medicine in Nuclear Medicine*, Proceedings of the 1992 Annual Hospital Information Management Systems Society (HIMSS) Conference, American Hospital Association, Chicago, Illinois.

Wilt, A. and Goddin, D. (1989), 'Health Care Case Study: Simulating Staffing Needs and Work Flow in an Outpatient Diagnostic Centre', *Industrial Engineering*, 21 (5), 22-26.

9 Strategy or Tactics? Technological Imperatives and Health Care Cost Control

JAMES R. SELDON[1] & GREG L. STODDART[2]

[1]*University College of the Cariboo, Canada*
[2]*McMaster University, Canada*

INTRODUCTION

Literature on the United States' health care cost crisis abound with references to technological origins. Similar concerns have been voiced world-wide. Aaron and Schwartz (1990) assert that technical change has been the single most important source of rising expenditures. Newhouse (1992) concludes that well over half of the 50-year increase in medical spending can be attributed to technological change. Evans (1984) contends that technology has defined medical need while capacity drives utilization. Weisbrod (1991: 524) argues that "insurance has paid for the development of cost-increasing technologies, and ... technologies have expanded demand for insurance." Fuchs (1986; 1990) criticizes recent innovation as cost-increasing. The common theme is that the benefits from technical advance have not justified the costs.

Static arguments focus on cost-increasing change and infatuation with sophisticated medical equipment. In a wry comment, Evans has quipped that there are more CT scanners than 7-Elevens in the United States.

One recurring complaint is that the acquisition and use of expensive technical apparatus is often driven by marketing rather than medical necessity. Unfortunately, the complainants rarely set their views of present outcomes against practicable alternatives, or spell out the precise nature of the putative resource misuse. Does competition for patients cause over-investment in medical research or result from it? Are individual practice styles overly capital-intensive and hence cost-ineffective; or are production patterns appropriate but output excessive? Is competition actually wasteful, or merely "unprofessional"? Since the various possibilities call for different remedies, work on specifics is warranted before policy can be directed at solutions. Even then, it is important to ask whether the outcome would be better or merely different.

Strategic Issues in Health Care Management. Edited by M. Malek, J. Rasquinha and P. Vacani
© 1993 John Wiley & Sons Ltd

Dynamic approaches typically focus on assertions that technical change has been biased toward cost-increasing techniques, although there are occasional claims that the rate of advance *per se* has been excessive. In either instance, advocates of intervention and control portray medico-technical advances creating demand and jobs while pushing up prices, costs and expenditures. The impression of technology spontaneously begetting demand is difficult to escape. Even Fuchs (1990), who takes pains to warn against blanket condemnation of technological change and who has long favoured less restrictive regulation of new pharmaceuticals (1974), nevertheless laments medical entrepreneurs developing and adopting *"any innovation that promised to improve the quality of care, regardless of cost."* (1990: 537, italics added)

The scenario of cost-increasing innovation often is coupled with pleas for more and better technology assessment or for more stringent application of 'need' standards. Thus, the relatively narrow, and perhaps broadly achievable, objective of cost-effectiveness is intertwined with the much more ambitious intent of ensuring economic (allocative) efficiency.

This paper's contention is that attention is diverted from substantive issues when technology is blamed for high or rising health expenditures. If patterns of resource use in health care are to be improved, focus must be on the gatekeepers and benefits, as well as the costs and must also be taken into account before judgements on the efficiency of resource use are pronounced.

TECHNOLOGY DOES NOT TREAT PEOPLE; PEOPLE TREAT PEOPLE

The rhetoric of spiralling costs and rising GDP shares sometimes hide obvious truths. One is that although technical change expands the boundaries of health care choice sets, neither practice styles nor utilization levels depend upon supply conditions alone.

Humans conceivably may possess utility functions embodying insatiable desires for improved health *states*. In practice, they show no tendency to demand, in economic not political terms, indefinitely large quantities of health *care*. (Even the staunchest opponents of universal health insurance in the United States appear to have given up on that particular bogey.) An important reason is that lowering direct charges to patients, even doing away with them, reduces the total price but by no means makes it zero. Point-of-service charges do not always appear in monetary terms, particularly with extensive insurance coverage, but search and inconvenience costs are just as real for those experiencing them. It follows that although extending insurance coverage will stimulate demand for health care, making its supply a more profitable enterprise and fostering investment in medical capital, the effect is finite and probably diminishing at the margin. Thus, even if extensions in insurance have played a major role in raising the share of resources flowing into health care; and even if the share is excessive; and even if production is overly capital-intensive, there still could be much to recommend benign neglect as a strategy for the future.

At one extreme, if markets for medical insurance, health care, and health care inputs were purely competitive and failure-free, technical change could be blamed for high or rising spending only in a largely trivial sense. It is instructive to examine innovation in this scenario before turning to the complexities of the real world.

In a perfectly competitive environment, resources would be directed to medical research if, and only if, their expected value was greater there than in available alternatives. "Expected" is an important qualifier. Hindsight inevitably would reveal cases in which alternative paths would have yielded higher returns, for even perfect markets cannot foretell the future more accurately than the collective prescience of their participants. There certainly could be lessons to be learned from what, with the clarity of hindsight, are revealed to have been "mistakes". However, there is no presumption that regulatory prescription or proscription would have improved affairs *ex ante* had they been substituted for the market's impersonal wisdom. Research is inherently risky, and the essence of decision-making in the presence of risk is that not all decisions can be expected to produce a positive return. Interventionists must demonstrate that their resource allocation decisions would be superior to those of the market, not merely that markets are imperfectly omniscient.

Ex post, with health care having become more effective (at whatever cost) and correcting for changes in other conditions (prices, incomes and preferences), knowledgeable consumers would bid to purchase more of it. Whether post-innovation spending rose, fell, or stayed the same, the effect always would be to raise social welfare as consumers responded to their new choice environments by once more voting with their dollars for the commodities they valued most highly. 'Errors' undoubtedly would occur. But again, they would only be wrong in hindsight.

The above discussion serves as a reminder that in competitive markets, constraining either buyers or sellers gives rise to outcomes failing the Paretian test. After accommodating all the constraints, there remain further changes in production and consumption patterns that are unachievable without removing the constraints, that could enhance the well-being of some members of society without doing harm to others. It is possible to conceive circumstances in which the social aggregate could be better off in such an arrangement than in the unconstrained competitive outcome. However, it is incumbent upon proponents of intervention to justify (case by case) the sacrifices they propose to levy on losers, the more so when it is not assured that there need be any winners.

Real-world health care markets at best are barely recognizable in the competitive prototype. Suppliers exercise monopoly power; consumers are ill-informed rather than ill, informed; and the agents employed to guide consumer choices have biases and opportunities of their own Despite lacking these attributes, the competitive case provides a useful baseline, and many of its conclusions are surprisingly robust.

Consider the effects of having individual producers possess monopoly power, whether as oligopolists or monopolistic competitors, when consumers are well-informed. Assume first that sellers successfully pursue maximum "profit" and that they are successful in their goal: their tactics involve underproducing and overcharging. Interventionist supply restrictions restraining the use of available production technology then further reduce output and cause the market price to rise yet higher. As in the competitive prototype, imperfectly competitive markets are moved away from their ideal performance when sellers are prevented from accommodating informed buyers. Since sellers must be operating on elastic portions of their individual demand curves, any one of them charging a higher price in isolation would find both gross and net earnings would fall. However, with inelastic aggregate demand for health care and all suppliers facing the same constraints, total expenditures will rise and providers will find themselves wealthier than before.

The fact that consumers are badly informed about health care's contribution to their health states seriously complicates the use of demand functions as value indicators but does not necessarily vitiate the above conclusions, as often seems to be taken for granted. Asymmetric information is a significant feature in health care, but it is important not to take its effects as self-evident. Geanakoplos (1992: 73) notes that "When it is common knowledge that agents are rational and optimizing, differences of information not only fail to generate a reason for trade on their own, but ... inhibit trade which would have taken place had there been symmetric information." Might the problem actually be that real-world markets generate too little health care, rather than too much? Again, the point is not that extra-market constraints on the use of technology are never appropriate, but that proposed interventions must be evaluated case by case.

If providers elect not to exploit their monopoly power for maximum financial gain, other possibilities emerge. Consider a setting in which providers adjust demand creation efforts to achieve target incomes. Interventionist supply restrictions, superimposed on constant demand creation effort and inelastic market demand, yield higher incomes. Higher incomes reduce the 'need' for demand creation. Lower demand creation offsets some of the price and expenditure increase. The ultimate impacts obviously depend on the objective functions of providers. If they strive for fixed target incomes and entry is barred, for instance, aggregate spending will be identical before and after the supply constraint is imposed. Fewer services will be supplied and fewer resources used than in the unconstrained initial case, but more than where firms are maximizing profit under similar circumstances. Whether an outcome is better or worse than in the unconstrained case again can only be determined case by case. If particular uses of technology are inappropriate, constraining them can yield benefits; but 'technology' is not the problem.

Externalities associated with new (or old) technology, saving costs in one arena at the cost of augmenting them elsewhere, constitute another potential justification for market intervention. Resource misallocation might be prevented by direct constraints on the development or use of a particular production technique, but a more attractive course of action might be to ensure that decision-makers evaluate the impact of each of their alternative choices would have.

It is easy to obtain consensus on the proposition that real-world markets for medical care are not perfectly competitive, and only somewhat more difficult to get broad agreement that market failure due to non control of monopoly power or externalities presents a *prima facie* case for intervention. However, the above discussion suggests that even those who are optimistic about the prospects for regulatory success will need more than the simple imperfections of real-world markets to justify controls over existing production techniques, let alone over research into new ones.

One approach to the latter prospect would be to argue that technical change, whether in pharmaceuticals, medical equipment, or surgical procedures, makes markets *more* imperfect: it accentuates problems brought on by asymmetric information and monopoly power, by making the connections between health care delivery and health status outcomes increasingly complex. Care is needed with this approach, but it does embody an important element of truth.

With efficacy and effectiveness difficult to assess, the value of accurate information, and the cost of error are both important. As technology becomes less comprehensible to patients and practitioners alike, the relative gap between efficiency and effectiveness widens as the practitioners find it profitable to invest in more and more specialized training. One implication is that new economies of scale and the expanded potential for exploitation of knowledge asymmetries by health care insiders strengthen the case for public rather than market-driven production and dissemination of information.

Government-administered technology assessment, coupled with controls such as Certificate of Need restrictions, may help to compensate for failure of the private market for information. However, when its focus is on cost effectiveness, technology assessment is a supply-side measure; the more difficult questions involve output values. Alone, effectiveness sheds little light on desirable levels of aggregate spending. Innovation is worthwhile when it causes spending in total to fall without reducing output; but it is no less so when value added more than offsets higher spending. The point again is simple but pivotal: *benefits as well as costs must be taken into account.*

The essential principle, is that spending on health care (private or public) is excessive only if the resources absorbed have higher-value uses elsewhere. One way of guarding against such excessive expenditures is to ensure that the choices of producers, consumers and agents all reflect the full costs and benefits of their actions. Banning goods from store shelves for the purpose of controlling middlemen is at best of dubious efficacy when there are both willing buyers and sellers, and if we are sufficiently well-informed to make those decisions, we can just as well implement appropriate tax and subsidy incentives.

The ultimate culprit in rising costs is not some abstraction called "technology", but human decision-makers on the demand and supply side of markets and institutions that supplement and substitute for markets. Even to the extent that growth in insurance coverage can be blamed for increased demand, it is well to recall that it is the motives and actions of individuals who determine the nature of institutions. Markets fail only when purposive behaviour leads to unintended consequences. A strategy designed to promote the most efficient use of scarce resources will only rarely be well served by tactics that involve denying market participants the opportunity to conclude what they see as mutually beneficial exchanges.

COST-SAVING MAY NOT SAVE COSTS

Intuition suggests that the distinction between cost-saving and cost-increasing technical change should be a meaningful one in debates over health care spending. The theme that policy might be directed at encouraging the former while constraining the latter is a common one.   Pharmaceuticals in particular earn kudos for cost reductions, despite occasional worries over pricing (The Economist, 1991) and fears of disasters such as thalidomide.   In contrast there is routine criticism of equipment such as scanners (which are overused because of excess capacity, and diagnose ailments of which patients would otherwise be blissfully ignorant) heart transplants and life-support systems (which prolong lives without curing').   Deeper thought reveals a rather more complex issue.

First, the effect of innovation on dollars spent, either absolutely or as shares of aggregate output, cannot tell the entire story.   If matters were that simple, computers, radial tyres, organically-grown foods and a host of other products would be the subject of concerned editorials citing fractions of GDP devoted to their production.   Instead, the relevant question is does the additional spending on new health technology generates greater value (including savings in costs that were hidden because they did not previously give rise to explicit cash transactions) than if it were utilised on other goods and services?.   Only if the answer is negative has the market failed to allocate resources to their optimal uses.

Second, effective technical change should make it possible to produce more output from a given quantity and quality of resource inputs.   Alternatively, technical change allows production of the same outputs as before but with lower input requirements.   It follows that the direct effects of *all* technical change, in health care as elsewhere, must be cost-*saving*.   Put another way, technical change involves the development of techniques that are more cost-effective than those currently in place. If total outlays are seen to increase following some medical innovation, the reason must be that the (quality-adjusted) volume of output has risen relatively faster than the cost per (standard-quality) unit has fallen.   Concerns over the higher flow of resources into medical care, then, must be directed not at overall input or output levels but at the opportunity foregone had the resources been utilised on some other programme more valuable to society.

In some instances, innovation can lead to a simple substitution of new production techniques for old, and to the attainment of original output levels at lower resource cost and lower monetary expenditures.   Bioengineering developments, yielding lower-cost production of insulin might fit this case.   There is little reason to expect that consumption would rise dramatically, even if the full savings were to be passed along in the form of lower prices, so that total cost would fall.   Technical change often allows for production of entirely new products and fosters higher total spending.   Again, consider a pharmaceutical advance, this time fostering a dramatic increase in the number of organ transplants in its ability to suppress tissue rejection. Whatever price is charged, it is apparent that a greater flow of resources will be drawn into health care to produce "new and improved" transplants.

Despite the cost-saving charms of the first example, benefits are clear, gains easily quantified and beneficiaries readily identified, versus the cost-increasing implications of the latter, it is important to recognize that from an economic perspective, neither is automatically superior. To further illustrate this point consider a choice between funding research on one or the other of the two drugs, and for simplicity assume the probability of a successful outcome are the same. If society places a high enough value on improved transplant capabilities, the preferred strategy tilts toward that research agenda despite its impact on health care spending. If there are great enough savings to be gained from lower-cost production of insulin which make this society's preferred area of resource expenditure, then the research agenda inclines to this direction.

Which alternative is better will depend upon whether market or other measures of costs and benefits are used in the evaluation, but the logic remains the same. No shorthand rule, such as observing total expenditures, can determine the best choice if it ignores the benefits side of the equation. The spending criterion may be popular because it is straightforward and easily applied. Alternatively, it may reflect lingering reliance on a "needs" model of medical care, where developments that free resources that can be devoted to other medical needs are preferable to those that threaten to absorb more resources. Whatever the reasons for its popularity, it will only by chance yield the right answers.

Third, recorded expenditure levels may or may not correctly measure or even proxy costs. Four outcomes are possible as a result of a change in technology: greater or lesser quantities of productive resources may flow to health care, and greater or lesser expenditure levels may accompany them. Consider a "cost-increasing" development in which the net effect of some innovation is to draw greater quantities of productive resources (land, labour, capital and entrepreneurial effort) into health care and away from other sectors of the economy. Slowing the pace of technical advance, or retarding adoption of extant technology, undeniably would restrict the resource flow, although as noted in Section II., it would also bid up prices and actually increase total spending on health care if market demand is inelastic. Since buyer spending equals supplier income, providers might well be grateful to policy-makers for exercising monopoly power on their behalf, but there can be no presumption that society as a whole would be well served. The restrictions would divert resources to lower-valued uses, hardly an obvious blueprint for welfare-enhancement. If, instead, demand were elastic, total expenditure would fall while prices rose, now spreading the harm between consumers and providers. There would be beneficiaries, those obtaining other commodities at lower prices because of the extra resources freed from producing health care, but the net effect would again be negative.

It might seem obvious that one would not wish to constrain "cost-saving" development. That conclusion follows as long as costs have been measured correctly and comprehensively, but the reasoning is as set out above, not the simplistic logic of cutting spending or saving resources. Thus, it does not follow that deliberate *promotion* of cost-saving ventures would be desirable unless there are hidden benefits not accounted for by market decision makers. Denying consumers the opportunity to obtain products they stand willing and able to pay for will make them worse off unless unusual circumstances govern the way in which resources are allocated. Inducing them to consume products they would reject were it not for a subsidy is similarly suspect.

CONCLUSION

This paper has argued that although technology is frequently blamed for rising health care expenditures, one set of concerns over the impact of innovation stems from misunderstanding costs while another flows from the tendency to ignore benefits. The contention is that the policies needed to promote efficient health care spending must be guided by more sophisticated reasoning than has often been evident even in the professional literature.

The overriding consideration is that *both* incremental costs *and* incremental benefits be taken into account when judgements on health care spending are being made. The most accurate cost-effectiveness measures in the world are useless if we cannot confirm that the output is of greater worth than alternative products the same inputs could generate. Technology assessment, structured to provide unbiased information on the links between inputs and outputs, is an essential aspect of the evaluation process, but it cannot shirk in its consideration of output values if it is to have any impact on expenditure decisions. Distinctions between cost-saving and cost-increasing innovation are meaningless for policy unless they are coupled with benefit measures.

"No one is arguing that technological innovation should slow down" runs a disclaimer (Garland 1991) of the sort accompanying many complaints about the rapid pace of change and the high cost of new technological achievement. However, that is precisely what many seem to infer. A case in point is Fuchs' (1983) warning that discovery of a costly cure for cancer would produce controversies over financing and selection of cases to be treated. Is not the message that society should withhold resources that might be devoted to the development of such a cure? (On the other hand, would not at least equally intense controversies attend the development and application of an inexpensive drug that euthanized patients suffering from incurable cancer, including some would have been restored to health by the new and expensive method not developed because of its cost implications?)

Fuchs (1990: 537) notes that "the character and magnitude of innovations in any particular sector are partly ... determined by demand emanating from the sector." Weisbrod (1991: 524) asserts that "long run growth of health care expenditures is a by-product of the interaction of the R & D process with the health care insurance system." The warnings are *a propos* for anyone wishing to understand the dynamics of health care supply and demand. However, endogeneity neither depends upon insurance coverage nor does provides justification for claims of excessive technical change.

Even if insurance does raise research efforts relative to a baseline scenario (certainly a plausible case) and even if the increased research leads to the development of medical technology that absorbs a larger share of society's resources, it is important to keep firmly in mind that increased spending is only undesirable if it involves directing resources to 'second-best' uses. When consumers insure themselves in anticipation of consuming more health care as a result, they are signalling their preferences and we ignore them at our peril.

In the end, we need to be suspicious of claims that "technology" is to blame for rising health care spending. First, spending is good or bad only in context. Unless we are truly on the flat of the (value) curve in health care, there can be no assurance that "less is better" until costs and benefits have been weighed. Second, it is difficult to accept the proposition that society should restrict research and development for fear of discovering what people might wish to spend their money on.

REFERENCES

Aaron, Henry J. and William B. Schwartz (1984), *The Painful Prescription: Rationing Hospital Care,* Brookings, Washington, D.C.

Aaron, Henry J. and William B. Schwartz (1990), 'Rationing Health Care: The Choice Before Us', *Science,* 247 (26 January), 418-422.

Carlisle, David M., A. L. Siu, E. B. Keeler, E. A. McGlynn, K. L. Kahn, L. V. Rubenstein and R. H. Brook (1992), 'HMO vs Fee-for-Service Care of Older Persons with Acute Myocardial Infarction', *American Journal of Public Health,* 82, 12 (December), 1626-1630.

The Economist (1991), 'Priceless Medicines', (26 October), 14-15.

Enthoven, Alain C. (1978), 'Cutting Cost Without Cutting Quality of Care', *New England Journal of Medicine,* 298 (22), 1224-1238.

Evans, Robert G. (1984), *Strained Mercy: The Economics of Canadian Health Care,* Butterworths, Toronto.

Feeny, David, G. Guyatt and P. Tugwell (1986), *Health Care Technology: Effectiveness, Efficiency and Public Policy,* Institute for Research on Public Policy, Montreal.

Fuchs, Victor (1983), *Who Shall Live? Health, Economics, and Social Choice,* Basic Books, New York.

Fuchs, Victor (1986), *The Health Economy,* Harvard: Cambridge, Mass.

Fuchs, Victor (1990), 'The Health Sector's Share of the Gross National Product', *Science,* 247 (2 February), 534-538.

Garland, Susan B. (1991), 'The Health Care Crisis: A Prescription for Reform', *Business Week,* 3234 (October 7), 58-66.

Geanakoplos, John (1992), 'Common Knowledge', *Journal of Economic Perspectives,* 6 (4), 53-82.

Newhouse, Joseph P. (1992), 'Medical Care Costs: How Much Welfare Loss?' *Journal of Economic Perspectives,* 6 (3), 3-22.

Weisbrod, Burton A. (1991), 'The Health Care Quadrilemma: An Essay on Technological Change, Insurance, Quality of Care, and Cost Containment', *Journal of Economic Literature*, 29 (June), 523-552.

Section III

National Standards and Performance Evaluation

10 Strategies for Improved Technology Assessment Use in European Health Care

ALA SZCZEPURA

University of Warwick

INTRODUCTION

Medical care is changing dramatically in all parts of the world; it is becoming more ambitious, more effective, but in the process also more expensive. Technology is regularly cited as a major contributor to the ever upward trend in health care costs in all western countries (Hoare 1992; Meyer 1990; Steering Committee on Future Health Scenarios 1987; OTA 1984; Jennett 1983). The term technology has a broad definition in health care. As the Office of Technology Assessment in the US defines it, health care technology is "the drugs, devices, and medical and surgical procedures used in medical care, and the organizational and support systems within which such care is delivered" (OTA 1978, 1982). All of the aspects which form an integral part of the delivery of health care.

Rising health care costs have sensitized health care decision-makers in both the private and the public sectors to the problems of scarce resources and multiple competing technologies (Oregon 1991; Dixon 1991; Australian Government 1990). Technological advances in medicine have been variously described as a "tidal wave" which threatens to overwhelm health care systems (Hoare 1992) or as a "driverless train running at increased speed towards an unknown destination" (Government Committee on Choices in Health Care 1992). In both these images it is the perceived lack of control, due to the absence of effective cost containment strategies, which is viewed as most threatening.

Health Care Technology Assessment (HTA) has gained increasing visibility during the 1980s and 1990s because of views such as these. HTA is the systematic process by which the direct and indirect consequences of a particular health care technology are assessed. It is concerned not only with the safety, quality, and effectiveness of health care technologies. Equally important are economic factors such as cost-effectiveness, and associated issues such as resource allocation and cost containment. The process of technology assessment incorporates a number of

Strategic Issues in Health Care Management. Edited by M. Malek, J. Rasquinha and P. Vacani
© 1993 John Wiley & Sons Ltd

distinct stages. Firstly, identification and selection of technologies which need to be assessed. Secondly, the design and performance of assessments. Thirdly, dissemination of results. Finally, incorporation of findings into decisions on use of these technologies. The ultimate aim of HTA is to inform policy-making and managerial and clinical decision-making in health care (Institute of Medicine 1985).

Many western governments have now set up formal mechanisms for the systematic assessment of health care technologies. In the USA, the Office of Technology Assessment was one of the front-runners in providing such technology assessment through a centralised approach (OTA 1984). Similar models are being introduced in Europe, although the number of experts in the field of HTA is relatively small and available centres of expertise often operate as individual 'enterprises' (Banta 1982; Blanpain 1983; Banta 1990). Increased co-ordination at the European level may in future go some way towards improving the use of scarce human resources in HTA.

The importance of HTA in European health care has been formally acknowledged. The WHO "Health For All" strategy, developed by the European Member States, included a commitment to implement 38 regional targets, the final one being:

• Target 38 - All Member States should have established a formal mechanism for the *systematic assessment* of the use of health technologies and of their effectiveness, efficiency, safety and acceptability.

The importance of HTA has been reiterated in a recent resolution of the Council and Ministers for Health (1991).

Although few would argue with the need for systematic technology assessment, there is no consensus on the most effective strategy for Europe (Banta 1990, Jonsson 1990; OECD 1990). It appears unlikely that any European country could mount a comprehensive HTA programme using the small number of academics and other experts currently active in the field. Therefore, one possible strategy might be to integrate HTA more effectively into the "business" of health care, both at the production end (medical technology industry) and at the user end (health care institutions) through encouraging a more systematic devolution of technology assessment to such organisations. Such a strategy will only succeed, however, if sufficient interest exists, or can be generated, in European organisations, and if appropriate skills are, or can be, made available within these organisations.

However, the current level and pattern of HTA interests in European organisations is largely unknown, as is their degree of expertise, and the extent to which they identify a need for HTA training. Therefore, research is urgently needed to explore the views of organisations involved in the production and use of technologies on their interests and need for expertise and competence in the area of health care technology assessment.

METHODOLOGY OF SURVEY

A survey was carried out covering a wide range of health care providers, health care funders, manufacturers, professional associations, academic institution, and policy making bodies in eight European countries. The survey was part of a much larger Project (COMETT-ASSESS). COMETT-ASSESS is funded by the EC and consists of a network of 35 universities, enterprises and health care organisations in 13 European countries, which have come together with the aim of improving the European base for health care technology assessment (COMETT-ASSESS 1993). COMETT-ASSESS is part of the second phase of COMETT - the European Community programme for co-operation between universities and industry for training in the field of technology. The aim of the COMETT programme is to reinforce training in order to develop highly skilled human resources and ensure the competitiveness of European industry. In health care, the term "industry" is not limited to manufacturers. It also includes health care providers such as hospitals, and purchasers of health care such as insurance and funding agencies.

Early in the COMETT-ASSESS Project it became evident that there is a lack of up-to-date information on existing HTA interests and training needs in Europe. It was therefore decided that a series of surveys would be carried out across a number of countries and organisations, in order to obtain information on:

- Existing levels of HTA interest and reasons for interest
- Existing levels of HTA expertise
- Areas in which organisations would like to improve their HTA competence and reasons why
- Types of staff who need training and the most appropriate forms of training

The survey covered a wide range of organisations involved in the production and use of health care technologies. Questionnaires were distributed over the period mid-1991 to mid-1992 by national representatives in seven different countries: Austria, Denmark, Finland, Germany, Ireland, Norway, and the United Kingdom. Each representative was asked to identify a mixture of organisations in approximately the following proportions: health care institutions (25%); professional associations (20%); industry or product manufacturers (15%); health care funding bodies or third-party payers (10%); policy making institutions (15%); and academic institutions (15%).

RESULTS

Nearly three hundred (288) organisations completed a detailed questionnaire about their HTA interests and training needs. The overall response rate was 19%; high for a postal survey of this type. The breakdown of respondents corresponded with the sampling frame set for the survey, although manufacturers were slightly over represented and professional associations somewhat under-represented. However, organisations could not always classify their role under one heading as requested; a significant number identified two or more functions for their organisation.

There was an even distribution between small-medium enterprises (56% of organisations reported less than 500 staff) and larger organisations (44% reported more than 500). Approximately one in three of the larger enterprises employed more than 5,000 staff. At a conservative estimate, the 288 organisations replying employ over 750,000 staff. Organisations were equally distributed between local, regional, national and international enterprises. The views represented in the survey should therefore not be biased in favour of organisations of a particular size, or those with a specific regional perspective.

Why Are Organisations Interested In HTA?

Organisations were asked why, if at all, they are interested in HTA, and asked to grade their *current level* of interest in selected aspects. The results demonstrate high levels of interest and also well defined reasons for this interest (Table 1). Organisations most frequently identified an interest in HTA because they want to improve "use of HTA in decision-making", and secondly to "improve general understanding of HTA". However, responses also demonstrate a high level of interest in designing and *performing HTA*; 91% of organisations reported such an interest, 44% rating it as high. There was far less interest in commissioning HTA from other agencies.

Table 1. Level of interest in different aspects of HTA (all respondents = 288)

Aspect of HTA	Level of interest			
	High 4-5	Med 3	Low 1-2	None 0
To perform HTA	44 %	20 %	28 %	9 %
To commission HTA	26 %	20 %	34 %	20 %
To use HTA in decision-making	53 %	25 %	19 %	3 %
To increase general understanding	50 %	28 %	21 %	1 %

A mean "score" for interest in these different aspects of HTA can be calculated from individual responses for a particular type of organisation (Table 2). The resulting scores show that different organisations all identify "improving use of HTA in decision-making" as their top priority.

In general, manufacturers report slightly lower scores, although their score for interest in "commissioning HTA" is the highest of any organisation. Health care institutions, on the other hand, exhibit the lowest interest score in commissioning assessments. Both types of organisation report a high score for interest in "performing HTA".

Health care providers and manufacturers are therefore both interested in initiating technology assessments, but it appears that providers would prefer to carry these out in-house, rather than commissioning them externally. This might be because many

Table 2. Mean score for interest in HTA — different organisations

Aspect of HTA	Mean score for differerent types of organisation						
	HC*	M*	PA*	AI*	RF*	PM*	Total
Performing HTA	3.1	3.0	2.8	2.9	3.2	2.6	2.9
Commisioning HTA	2.3	2.8	2.5	2.6	2.6	2.3	2.3
Using HTA in decision-making	3.4	3.3	3.4	3.7	3.6	3.5	3.4
Increasing general understanding	3.4	3.2	3.3	3.7	3.3	3.3	3.3

* Type of organisation: HC= Health care institution; M= Industry/ manufacturer;
PA= Professional association; AI= Academic institution;
RF= Health care reimbursement/ funding agency; PM= Policy making institution/ agency

European health care institutions already have sufficient internal expertise to design and carry out technology assessments.

Manufacturers, on the other hand, are as interested in commissioning assessments as they are in carrying them out in-house. This might imply lower levels of in-house expertise than health care providers, and a resulting need to use external skills.

Finally, health care reimbursement and funding agencies report the greatest interest in performing technology assessments. Once again, it is not clear to what degree this is linked to high levels of existing HTA expertise in these organisations. They also report a high level of interest in commissioning HTA from external agencies.

When Should Technologies Be Assessed?

Organisations were asked to indicate their level of interest in technology assessment at different points in the life cycle of a technology; these included emerging technologies (i.e. those not yet fully developed), new technologies (i.e. those recently introduced), and accepted technologies (i.e. technologies in widespread use). Respondents as a whole reported highest interest in assessment of *new* technologies, and the second highest in assessment of *accepted* ones. The lowest reported interest was in *emerging* technologies.

These views differed depending on the type of organisation. Organisations show most interest in assessment of technologies which directly affect their efficiency, effectiveness or profitability.

For manufacturers, interest is focused on *new* technologies i.e. ones which have just entered the market. For health care institutions and health care funding agencies, although they similarly reported high levels of interest in assessment of *new* technologies, their interest in *accepted* technologies is equal or even higher. Interest in *emerging* technologies is relatively low. The pattern reported by health care providers and funders contrasts sharply with the main emphasis in many technology assessment programmes on emerging or new technologies, often to the exclusion of accepted technologies where there may be a tacit understanding that it is too late for technology assessment. The survey findings therefore provide worrying indications that HTA programmes may not be meeting the needs of these organisations.

When an organisation's interest in HTA at specific points of the technology life cycle was compared with their reasons for interest in HTA, it was found that organisations with a high level of interest in *performing HTA* reported high levels of interest in assessment of new and accepted technologies, and much less interest in emerging technologies.   On the other hand, organisations interested in *commissioning HTA* reported most interest in new technologies, and equal (but much lower) interest in emerging and accepted ones.

A relationship between interest in commissioning and interest in assessment of emerging technologies is not unexpected; this is consistent with the content of much commissioned research.   However, the second pattern is more interesting; a relationship between a desire to perform HTA and an interest in assessment of accepted technologies.   This may indicate that organisations contemplating a "do-it-yourself" approach are doing so because existing assessment programmes do not meet their needs in this area.   Assessment of accepted technologies may therefore provide an effective mechanism for initial devolution of HTA, especially if accepted technologies continue to be excluded from most main stream HTA programmes.

Which Technologies Are Of Interest?

Finally, organisations were asked to identify the types of health care technologies which are of most importance or interest to them.   The responses here show that the most widespread interest is currently in information systems (particularly clinical systems) and pharmaceuticals, with therapeutic technologies and diagnostics coming next.   This pattern varies somewhat depending on the type of organisation. Manufacturers report a fairly *narrow* spectrum of technology interests which primarily focuses on technologies that they market themselves, although respondents did show a higher level of interest than anticipated in certain technologies, particularly clinical information systems (55% interested whereas only 13% were IT manufacturers).   In sharp contrast, organisations involved in the delivery or funding of health care are interested in an extremely *wide* range of health care technologies. This is also true for health care policy makers, and to a slightly lesser extent professional associations and academic institutions.

A Framework for Competence in Technology Assessment

Although considerable effort has been devoted in recent years to defining competence in a wide range of technical, clinical, and managerial areas, at the time of writing, there is still no internationally accepted framework for competence in HTA. In order to identify HTA training needs, the study had therefore first to define such a framework.   An international panel of experts in HTA was used to identify possible areas, or elements, of HTA competence.   Initial discussions produced consensus on 59 elements.   These were then structured into 13 'domains'.   The objective was to construct domains which were internally consistent, reasonably self-contained, and which could form the basis of a sensible training programme.   The initial list was circulated to national representatives in all member countries and an amended version produced, which was then circulated for final agreement; a form of Delphi Technique (Jewell 1981). In this way a number of domains and associated outcome competencies were identified for use in the survey (table 3).

Table 3. HTA domains used in survey

Domain Number	Definition	Outcome competence
1	Language definitions of HTA	*staff able to understand and use appropriate; HTA language and definitions*
2	Background to HTA	*staff able to understand origins of HTA and current status*
3	Methodologies for HTA	*staff competent to understand a range of basic HTA methodologies*
4	Which method to use	*staff competent to identify the most appropriate methodology for particular situation / requirement*
5	HTA versus life cycle	*staff competent to understand technology diffusion and advantages of HTA at different stages in life cycle*
6	Outcome measures for HTA	*staff competent to identify and use appropriate outcome measures for use in HTA*
7	Organising/running HTA	*staff competent to successfully organise and run HTA*
8	How to interpret/critique HTA	*staff competent to evaluate study methodology, timing, results and possible impact of HTA results*
9	Implementing HTA findings	*staff competent to implement findings and aware of challenges and opportunities in implementation*
10	Clinical practice and HTA	*staff competent to understand how HTA results might influence clinical practice*
11	HTA and product development	*staff competent to understand role of industry in HTA, and how HTA can affect product development*
12	HTA and health policy	*staff competent to understand the developing relationship between HTA and health policy*
13	Funding for HTA	*staff competent to identify issues related to funding of HTA*

The domains form a hierarchy, ranging from expertise in "language and definitions of HTA" through to the ability to "organise and run HTA", and finally competence in "implementing HTA findings". In addition, further domains were included which it was considered might prove to be organisation-specific; for example, "clinical practice and HTA" for those involved in providing or funding health care, "HTA and product development" which might be mainly of interest to manufacturers, "HTA and health policy" to policy makers, and "funding for HTA" of interest to health care funding organisations.

European HTA Training Needs

Organisations were asked to grade their current level of expertise in each of the thirteen domains on a 1-5 scale. Next, they were asked to grade the *value* to their organisation of expertise in these same domains. A glossary sheet was provided explaining the content of each domain.

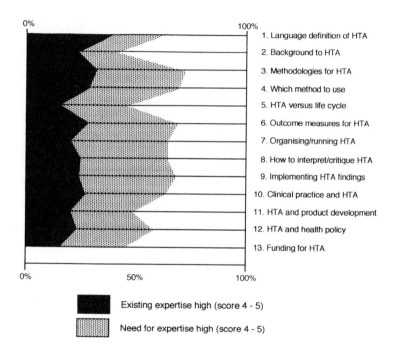

Figure 1. Percentage of respondents grading existing expertise, or need of expertise as high. Existing HTA expertise and need for expertise , all respondents (n = 228)

The overall pattern of responses, for all organisations surveyed, is shown in Figure 1. This displays the percentage of organisations who reported a high level of existing expertise (score 4-5), juxtaposed against the percentage who attached a similarly high level of importance to expertise in that domain. The dark shaded profile to the left can therefore be considered to represent the existing level of expertise; the profile to the right represents the importance attached to expertise in each domain; the dotted area remaining represents the "shortfall" in expertise. Clearly, European organisations currently report substantial shortfalls in HTA expertise for all 13 domains. This shortfall (M) can be quantified for an individual organisation:

$$M = \text{(Level of Importance of Expertise)} - \text{(Level of Existing Expertise)}$$

If the value of M is positive, this indicates a shortage of expertise; if it is zero or negative, there is sufficient or excess expertise. The mean value of M can then be calculated across a group of respondents to give a quantitative measure of the level of mismatch in the group. Mean values of M are displayed in Figure 2 for the group as a whole.

Figures 1 and 2 illustrate that skills shortfalls are lowest in domains such as "language and definitions of HTA" and "background to HTA" which occur early in the hierarchy. Much larger shortfalls are reported in later domains, linked to *applied* skills such as those of designing and running HTA studies, or the skills needed to implement HTA findings.

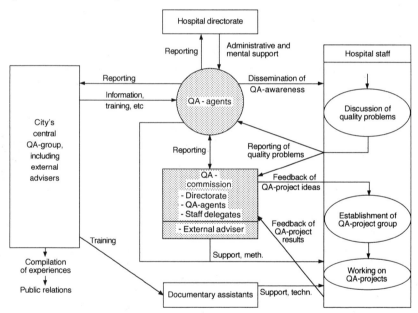

Figure 2. Mismatch (M) between level of expertise and importance of expertise. Existing HTA expertise and need for expertise , all respondents (n = 228)

Variations Between Organisations

The shortfall, or perceived training need, in an organisation will depend both on existing skills levels and on the value placed on competence. Both of these may vary depending on the type of organisation.

Health care institutions are found to report the largest training needs, particularly acute in practical domains associated with performing assessments and implementing HTA findings. It has already been shown these organisations exhibit the greatest interest in performing technology assessments. Clearly, the desire to perform HTA is not at present complemented by sufficient competence in organising and running assessments. Similarly, other organisations who reported a high level of interest in performing HTA (eg manufacturers and health care funding agencies) currently gauge their practical expertise as fairly low.

Manufacturers generally place a slightly lower value on expertise in many HTA domains than do other organisations. This, combined with fairly high levels of existing expertise, results in the lowest competence shortfalls being observed in this group. Furthermore, the pattern of shortfalls which they reveal differs from those of most other organisations. For example, HTA and product development is the greatest training need among manufacturers, with improved competence in organising and running assessments of only secondary importance. These are followed by a need to increase expertise in interpreting and critiquing HTA (perhaps linked to the interest which manufacturers report in commissioning HTA studies), and also a need to improve understanding of the relationship between HTA and health policy.

Reimbursement and funding agencies similarly report fairly high levels of existing expertise, resulting in the lowest competence shortfall after manufacturers. However, although their interest profile is very similar to that of manufacturers, their major training needs are in clinically-related areas such as outcome measures, and HTA and clinical practice. In this respect they turn out to be very similar to professional associations.

Academic institutions also report quite high levels of existing expertise (almost as high as manufacturers). Furthermore, they perceive their main training needs in areas such as methodologies and choice of method, funding for HTA, and HTA and health policy. They clearly report less need to increase competence in organising and running HTA, or in critiquing and interpreting HTA studies.

Professional associations on the other hand, are similar to health care institutions in that they have relatively low levels of existing expertise and place a relatively high value on improved competence. However, the focus of their training needs is less on performing HTA, and more on what comes next; implementing HTA findings, outcome measures, clinical practice and HTA, as well as the skills of interpreting and critiquing HTA studies, and improved understanding of HTA and health policy.

Finally, policy makers exhibit a profile which is very similar to that reported by health care institutions. Their level of existing expertise turns out to be low, with major mismatches in identical areas, except that funding for HTA is now identified as an important training need.

Table 4 provides an overview of the various organisations surveyed. Generally, for all types of organisations training needs are less evident (L) in domains such as language and definitions of HTA and background to HTA. Similarly, all organisations (except manufacturers) report little training need in HTA and product development; for manufacturers, however, this is the top training need. When the areas in which major skills shortages exist (H) are considered, patterns are slightly less clear cut. Although much of the training need is in practical areas such as deciding which HTA method to use, organising and running HTA and implementing

Table 4. Skills shortfalls reported by different organisations

Domain	Definition	Type* of Organisation					
		HCI	M	PA	AI	RF	PM
1	Language definition of HTA	L*	L			L	L
2	Background to HTA	L	L	L	L	L	L
3	Methodologies for HTA	H*			H	H	H
4	Which method to use	H			H		H
5	HTA versus life cycle		L	L	L		
6	Outcome measures for HTA			H		H	
7	Organising/running HTA	H	H				H
8	How to interpret/critique HTA		H	H			
9	Implementing HTA findings	H		H			H
10	Clinical practice and HTA			H		H	
11	HTA & product development	L	H	L	L	L	L
12	HTA and health policy		H	H	H	H	
13	Funding for HTA				H		H

*L = One of lowest training needs identified;
 H = One of highest training needs identified

HTA findings, methodologies for HTA and HTA and health policy also figure prominently as key training needs.

Who Needs Training?

Having identified an extensive range of training needs, it was necessary to consider the feasibility of meeting these. In order to answer this question, all organisations were asked to identify up to three key target groups for training. The majority of organisations (51%-60%) identified a select number of staff (less than 10) in each target group. Only a small percentage of respondents (15-16%) identified target groups of more than 90.

Virtually all organisations (92%) were able to identify at least one target group, 85% identified two groups, and approximately half (55%) identified three. The two types of staff most frequently identified were managers (77% of organisations) and clinicians (66%). Other personnel, such as researchers and marketing staff, generally formed a lower priority for training. Company trainers themselves featured very low on the list of priorities; most organisations did not identify these staff until asked to select their third target group.

Results show that the staff requiring training differ depending on the type of organisation. Health care institutions almost exclusively identify clinicians and managers as their target groups for training, with a greater emphasis on researchers in their second target group, and trainers in their third. Manufacturers on the other hand identify managers and marketing staff as their primary target groups, and researchers (or managers) as their second. In contrast, professional associations and academic institutions pick out clinicians and researchers. Finally, health care funding agencies and policy makers both identify clinicians as most important in their first target group, researchers in their second, and trainers in their third.

Why Do Staff Need Training?

When asked why staff need training, it is observed that the highest priority in all organisations is to improve their decision-making abilities; followed by increased competence in design and performance of assessments and improved general understanding with improved criticizm of HTA studies, being the least important priority..

This pattern changes slightly for different staff groups. Managers principally need training to be able to use HTA information in their decision-making (69%), and secondly, to improve general understanding. A similar pattern emerges for marketing staff (71% for decision-making). Research staff mostly need training to improve their ability to design and perform HTA (57%), and secondly, to commission technology assessments (32%). Clinicians principally need to improve their use of HTA in decision-making (58%), and secondly to improve their ability to design and perform HTA (31%). Finally, trainers principally need training to improve their general understanding of HTA (57%).

What Form of Training?

When asked to identify suitable forms of training, the majority of organisations identified a number of possible options for each target group (Table 5). In general, it is apparent that organisations would prefer either short (2-3 day), intensive, external workshops or training within the organisation by consultants. Both forms of training clearly differ from the more usual academic, full-time courses offered by many educational establishments. Full-time courses of this type are considered appropriate by fewer than one in five organisations. In addition, only two types of organisations showed significant interest in distance learning; professional associations (17%) and academic institutions (20%). In the case of professional associations, this may be because their target groups were generally larger (one in three reported groups larger than 90), which will make this form of learning more attractive. Professional associations also reported the highest level of interest in computer assisted learning (12%).

The two preferred forms of training should offer rapid training with minimum disruption to the organisation. They might be especially suitable if key individuals cannot be removed from the organisation for long periods. Analysis supports this view. It shows that managers, marketing staff and clinicians figure prominently in this group. Full-time courses are mainly identified as appropriate for other staff such as researchers and trainers.

The desire for rapid training is even more apparent when organisations were asked to estimate the total length of training required. Seven out of ten organisations judged that an individual could be trained within 5 days overall. This might appear overly optimistic, but once again it was staff such as managers, clinicians, and marketing personnel who were included in this group; more extensive training was judged to be appropriate for researchers and trainers.

Table 5. What type of training is suitable for different organisations?

Definition	Percentage of 3 target groups					
	HCI	M	PA	AI	RF	PM
Outside organisation						
2 - 3 day workshops	41	41	32	29	43	48
Full - time course	18	22	18	22	11	22
Inside organisation						
Company trainers	20	21	24	25	21	16
Consultants	37	30	35	25	46	42
Alternative forms						
Distance / self	13	17	14	20	10	14
CAL*	9	12	6	9	6	11
Other methods	4	9	8	5	5	2

*computer assisted learning

Turning to the learning sets within which individuals should receive training, most organisations identified a need for mixed staff groups or disciplines; only one in three considered this inappropriate. Responses were similar regardless of the type of organisation, but they did vary somewhat with the type of staff group; mixed learning sets were considered least suitable for researchers and trainers.

When asked about the scale on which HTA training should be provided, the majority of organisations selected national or international level (two out of three). International training was most highly favoured by manufacturers (45%), and national training by professional associations (54%). The desire for larger scale training and mixed participant groups both support an image of HTA as transcending professional and national boundaries.

DISCUSSION

It is certain that advances in medical technology will continue to increase the gap between health care which can be provided within available budgets, and health care which could be provided if there were no financial constraints (Feeny 1986; Banta 1990; Dixon 1991). Choices will therefore need to be made about which health care technologies are made available, and their conditions of availability (OTA 1985; Hiatt 1987; Drummond 1987; Stocking 1988; Szczepura 1992a). Health care is fast entering an age in which new technologies will no longer be introduced, or perhaps even marketed, without some form of prior assessment. At the same time, existing technologies may also need to be closely scrutinised. At present few decisions over the development, introduction, or discontinuation of medical technologies are made in such an informed way. The number of new technologies which European health care might need to assess in the coming decade is extremely large (Steering Committee on Future Health Scenarios 1987; Hoare 1992), and the task is even more daunting if assessment of existing technologies is also to be included. This clearly raises the question of which technologies should be assessed.

At present the major emphasis in many HTA programmes is on technologies before they enter the general service setting (emerging or new technologies). This is partly because more rigorous methodologies (such as randomised controlled trials) can be used before any widespread "acceptance", and also because there are distinct advantages for policy makers and reimbursement agencies in encouraging assessment prior to such widespread diffusion. In contrast, the present survey results show that European organisations are more interested in assessment of *accepted* technologies than emerging ones, especially policy makers and funding agencies. Therefore, HTA programmes which focus on emerging technologies are likely to fail to meet this important need. More thought therefore needs to be given to developing methodologies for assessing technologies once they have reached the service setting (Szczepura 1992b). The survey responses also show that organisations consistently report highest interest in technologies whose end product is information (eg information systems, medical imaging and other diagnostics). To date, much HTA has focused on technologies with a *direct* impact on patients (eg pharmaceuticals and clinical procedures) rather than grappling with the more difficult challenge of technologies whose main product is information (either clinical or managerial). This is especially true if these technologies are also likely to change with advances in software eg IT systems, medical imaging (Institute of Medicine 1991; Szczepura 1991). Major effort now needs to be invested in developing appropriate methodologies for use with such "moving target" technologies.

The second major challenge in HTA is ensuring the effective use of assessment findings. There is little point in conducting detailed technology assessments if the resulting information is not used. To date, one of the main influences on the development of HTA has been the desire to ensure its acceptance as an academic discipline. Methodologies for assessing health care technologies, production of scientifically rigorous HTA results, and publication in academic journals have therefore taken precedence. Far less effort has been devoted to ensuring that, once published, HTA information is effective in improving European health care.

Government bodies and national insurance agencies have been the first to appreciate the potential value of HTA information. But, it appears that HTA findings are still little used at a lower organisational level, especially by managers and clinicians. Up to now the consensus has been that this is mainly due to lack of awareness, and efforts are now being made in many countries to disseminate HTA findings more widely (Department of Health 1992).

However, the results of the present study raise fundamental questions about the validity of such a conclusion. Responses show that, far from being unaware of the possible value of HTA, a wide range of European organisations already understand its potential importance. More than 95% of survey respondents want to increase their use of HTA information in decision-making, a similar percentage to increase general understanding of HTA, and nine out of ten would now like to perform technology assessments.

But, high levels of interest are not matched by comparably high levels of competence. When questioned (using a hierarchy of HTA competencies defined for the first time in this study) all types of organisations consistently report extensive training needs in a number of key areas. For all organisations, when asked why training is needed, the main reason given is to improve use of HTA findings in decision-making. This illustrates the importance of developing effective training strategies in conjunction with any HTA dissemination initiatives, if HTA findings are to be used more effectively by decision-makers.

In addition to a desire to improve use of HTA findings in decision-making, the survey responses also indicate that a majority of organisations (six out of ten) also want to train staff to design and perform assessments. Three types of organisation expressed most interest in this; health care institutions, manufacturers, and reimbursement or funding agencies. However, responses also show that the organisations with the highest level of interest in performing HTA (health care institutions) currently report the lowest levels of existing HTA expertise. The largest training needs therefore exist in those organisations which are most keen to become actively involved in HTA.

The future of HTA in Europe will ultimately be shaped by existing interest in HTA, levels of expertise in organisations, and the extent to organisations want to improve their HTA knowledge and skills. At the technology user end, it appears likely that health care institutions will become increasingly aware of the need for HTA as they are faced with the task of containing costs while maximising effectiveness and health gain. Similarly, reimbursement or health care funding agencies (who are the ultimate purchasers of health care technologies) are certain to develop an increased interest in HTA if they consider it can help to maximise effective use of scarce resources. At the other end of the spectrum (the manufacturer end), it seems likely that European industries will exhibit increased interest in HTA for a variety of reasons. Firstly, because health care cost containment strategies introduced by governments in other parts of the world (such as Australia and Canada) may soon start to appear in Europe. If they do, these will require manufacturers to provide information on the cost-effectiveness of new health product (especially pharmaceuticals) as well as on their safety and efficacy (Drummond 1992; Government Committee on Choice in Health Care 1992; Institute of Medicine 1991). Secondly, if *purchasers* of medical technologies become more knowledgeable about HTA, manufacturers may need to incorporate technology assessments into the development of most new products, both because the financial risk of unsuitable research investments and inappropriate production decisions will be too high otherwise, and also because it will improve market potential.

In the 1990s, the success of European HTA strategies will depend on the roles which different types of organisations are prepared to adopt. This will also naturally have an impact on their training needs. If organisations consider that technology assessments should continue to be largely designed and carried out by others, they may view themselves primarily as end-users of HTA information. In this case, their major training need will be to improve their use of HTA findings in decision-making.

Alternatively, organisations may also wish to improve their skills in commissioning technology assessments, in which case they presumably hope to have some influence on the technologies chosen for assessment but little on assessment methodologies, and no direct involvement in assessment itself. Finally, organisations may identify a need to train their staff to design and carry out technology assessments. In this case, they clearly foresee an active role for themselves in any European HTA strategy.

Organisations which are interested in performing HTA should prove of immense value in the 1990s, if they are also competent to design and perform assessments. It is likely that increasing numbers of technologies will need to be assessed during the decade, especially if government policies enforcing assessment of new health care products prior to licensing become widespread. In comparison to the size of the task, the number of experts currently active in the field of HTA and those being trained is very small. Urgent consideration now needs to be given to developing a European training strategy to meet the needs of organisations who express an interest in performing technology assessments.

CONCLUSIONS

The study findings raise several important questions, many of which call for urgent attention and action from policy makers and senior management. Included among these are questions about the types of technologies which should be being assessed, the need to integrate HTA training with dissemination of assessment findings so that better use is made of HTA results in decision-making, and the need to provide appropriate training in the design and performance of assessments so that more cost-effective strategies can be developed for comprehensive technology assessment in Europe.

REFERENCES

Australian Government (1990), *Discussion paper on ethics and resource allocation in health care*, Australian Government Publishing Service, Canberra.

Banta H D, Kemp K (eds) (1982),*The management of health care technology in nine countries*, Springer Publishing Company, New York.

Banta H D, Andreasen P B (1990), 'The political dimension in health care technology assessment', *International Journal of Technology Assessment in Health Care*, 6, 115-123.

Blanpain J E (1983), Health technology assessment in Belgium, France, Germany and Japan, Acta Hospitilia, 23 p37.

COMETT-ASSESS (1993 Forthcoming), *Final Report of the COMETT-ASSESS Project*, J Kankaanpaa, Helsinki, Finland.

Council and Ministers for Health, Resolution of the Council, Brussels November 7th, 1991, concerning fundamental health policy choices (91/C 304/05)

Department of Health (1992), *Assessing the Effects of Health Technologies: Principles, Practice, Proposals*, Department of Health, London.

Dixon J, Gilbert Welch H (1991), 'Priority Setting: lessons from Oregon', *The Lancet*, 337, 891-94.

Drummond M (1987), 'Economic evaluation and the rational diffusion and use of health technology', *Health Policy*, 7, 309-324.

Drummond M (1992), 'Economic evaluation of pharmaceuticals - Science or marketing?', *Pharmaco Economics* 1: 8-13.

Feeny D, Guyatt G, Tugwell P (1986), *Health care technology: effectiveness, efficiency & public money*, The Institute for Research on Public Policy, Montreal.

Government Committee on Choices in Health Care (1992), *Choices in Health Care*, Ministry of Welfare, Health and Cultural Affairs, Rijswijk, The Netherlands

Hiatt H H (1987), 'Advances in Medical Technology' in *America's Health in Balance*, Harper & Row, New York, 49-68.

Hoare J (ed) (1992) *Tidal Wave: New Technology, Medicine and the NHS*, King's Fund Centre, London.

Institute of Medicine (1985), *Assessing Medical Technologies*, Report of the Committee for Evaluating Medical Technologies in Clinical Use, National Academic Press, Washington DC.

Institute of Medicine (1991), *The Changing Economics of Medical Technology*, AC Gelijns and EA Halm (ed), National Academic Press, Washington DC.

Jennett B (1983), High technology medicine, benefits and burdens, The Nuffield Provincial Hospitals Trust, London.

Jewell L N and Reitz H J (1981), *Group Effectiveness in Organisations*, Illinois: Scott, Foresman, Glenview.

Jonsson B, Rutten P, Vang J (eds) (1990), *Policy making in health care: Changing goals and new tools*, Linkoping University.

Meyer J et al (1990), *Critical Choices, confronting the costs of American health care*, Report to the National Committee for Quality of Health Care, Washington DC.

OECD (1990), *Health care in transition*, OECD Social Policy Studies No 7, Paris.

Oregon-report (1991), Health Services Commission, Oregon, USA.

OTA: Office of Technology Assessment (1978), *Assessing the efficacy and safety of medical technologies*, Washington DC: US Government Printing Office.

OTA: Office of Technology Assessment (1982), *Strategies for medical technology assessment*, Washington DC: US Government Printing Office.

OTA: Office of Technology Assessment (1984), *Medical technology and costs of the Medicare program*, Washington DC: US Government Printing Office, 41-53.

OTA: Office of Technology Assessment (1985), *Medicare's prospective payment system: Strategies for evaluating cost, quality, and medical technology*, Washington DC: US Government Printing Office.

Steering Committee on Future Health Scenarios (1987), *Anticipating and Assessing Health Care Technology*, Volume 1. General considerations and policy conclusions, Martinus, Nijhoff Publishers, Dordrecht, The Netherlands

Stocking B (1988), 'Medical technology in the United Kingdom', *International Journal of Technology Assessment in Health Care*, 4, 171-83.

Szczepura A K, Fletcher J, Fitz-Patrick J D (1991), 'Cost effectiveness of magnetic resonance imaging in the neurosciences', *British Medical Journal*, 303, 1435-1439.

Szczepura A K (1992a), 'Rush to Arms; how cost-effective are new additions to the clinician's armoury?' *The Health Service Journal*, 102;5286, 20-22.

Szczepura A K (1992b), 'Routine low cost pathology tests; measuring the value-in-use of bacteriology tests in hospitals and primary care', *Health Services Management Research*, 5; 225-237.

11 Customer Supplier Modelling as a Framework for Quality Improvement

VICTORIA DOYLE[1,2], EWART CARSON[1,2] & PETER SÖNKSEN[2,1]

[1]*City University, London*
[2]*St Thomas' Hospital, London*

QUALITY IN HEALTH CARE

Concern about the quality of health care has stimulated a huge array of initiatives which have affected primary and tertiary care country-wide (Moss 1992). Implementation of formal mechanisms for ensuring the quality of patient care is recognised as an important goal by the NHS for this decade (DoH 1989; Relman 1988).

The rationale of quality improvement is to create an environment where it is possible to understand and be responsive to patient needs. For this to happen regular, critical and systematic analysis and evaluation of clinical practice is required (DoH 1989). This must include the contributions to care given by all professional groups and take in both the clinical and non-clinical aspects of the health care system. Though guidelines, protocols and standards of care have been developed by professional groups for specific problems, comprehensive guidelines covering several levels of care (from primary to tertiary) and several provider groups are rare (Vuori 1992). Much good quality care is dependent on collaboration and communication between these provider groups. Now that audit of clinical practice is becoming established and accepted, a framework for coherent, interdisciplinary audit is required, bringing together all the quality initiatives. Otherwise it is very likely that these different initiatives will become isolated, ineffectual activities (Moss 1992).

This paper sets out to show how it is possible to bring the different provider groups together and create a framework for interdisciplinary audit and quality improvement. The approach adopted to achieve this end is customer supplier modelling, a technique which originated from industry (Doyle *et al* 1992).

Strategic Issues in Health Care Management. Edited by M. Malek, J. Rasquinha and P. Vacani
© 1993 John Wiley & Sons Ltd

CUSTOMER SUPPLIER RELATIONSHIPS

The customer supplier relationship is an important tenet of the Total Quality Management philosophy (Oakland 1989). The emphasis is on external customers or recipients of care, in that all that is done is done for the benefit of the patient. However it is also important to be aware of the internal customer supplier relationships that exist within all organisations. The work of individuals and departments within health care organisations are interconnected. As such people and departments act as their own internal 'suppliers' and 'customers' and it is their interconnected activities which are intended to benefit the external customer (Lohr 1990).

Figure 1 describes a simple customer supplier relationship. The supplier is a person or unit which supplies a product or service as requested by the customer. The supplier is also responsible for the design and operation of that product or service. The customer is the person or unit who requests the product or service and/or is the person who uses or consumes that product or service. Both supplier and customer have their own expectations of that service or product and normally there is a form of dialogue between customer and supplier to understand these needs. This should be a two way exchange of information.

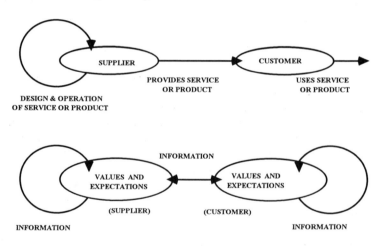

Figure 1. Customer supplier relationship

CUSTOMER-SUPPLIER MODELLING

Even in the most simple of transactions, there is very rarely only one supplier and customer involved. In more complex clinical practice there tends to be many different customers and suppliers in order to satisfy one operation. This results in the formation of a customer supplier model, which is in effect a series of single customer supplier relationships linked together. This modelling technique can be used to describe the activities of a person, speciality, directorate or unit. To detail the operational and clinical activities of one of these categories it must include all the different provider groups involved in delivering that specific service.   Thus the technique can provide the framework for bringing the different provider groups together and also provide a degree of coherency for their audit activities.

Figure 2 gives an example of a customer supplier model. The model shows the different customers and suppliers involved when ordering a diagnostic test (eg a Mid Stream Urine test) and its results. The focus of this model is the diabetes day centre which is the main provider of care for the patient. The patient is described as an internal customer, since the referral to the day centre has already been made. Microbiology is labelled as an external department, because it is not an integral part of the day centre. The customer supplier relationships, numbered from one to six show the various stages of delivering this service.

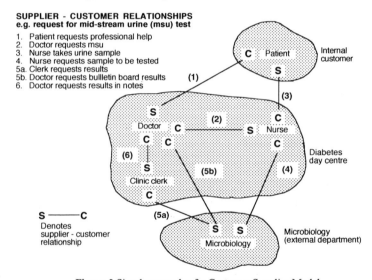

SUPPLIER - CUSTOMER RELATIONSHIPS
e.g. request for mid-stream urine (msu) test

1. Patient requests professional help
2. Doctor requests msu
3. Nurse takes urine sample
4. Nurse requests sample to be tested
5a. Clerk requests results
5b. Doctor requests bullletin board results
6. Doctor requests results in notes

Figure 2.Simple example of a Customer Supplier Model

This methodology of customer-supplier modelling can be extended to the entire Health Care Model (figure 3) which shows the interactions between the different actions involved in the system as a whole.

When attempting to model the activities of a group it is important to consider group culture which is made up of the behaviour, actions and attitudes of its members (Schein 1987). This group culture is developed as the group learns to cope with problems of external adaptation and internal integration. Therefore the customer-supplier modelling process is divided into two quite separate parts. These are 'external adaptation modelling' and 'internal integration modelling'. The former process describes how the group work and adapt with other people. This involves pin-pointing the external bodies which have an influence over and active involvement in the way a particular group of carers operate and deliver health care. These external

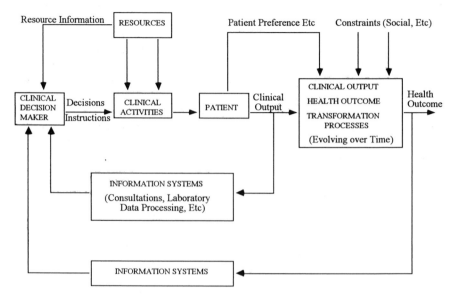

Figure 3. The overall health care model

bodies may be suppliers, customers or both. The latter process involves defining quite explicitly how the group work and integrate together. This is describing how they act as suppliers and customers to each other.

Thus external adaptation modelling is concerned with how services, products and people interface with or enter the group, whereas internal integration modelling is concerned with what actually happens within the group.

PILOT DEPARTMENTAL MODELLING APPROACH

This modelling technique is being used and refined at St Thomas' Hospital, London in two different departments:

- gynaecological in-patient ward
- diabetes day centre

An in-patient and out-patient setting were selected to show that this technique is equally applicable in different clinical settings. A departmental approach was chosen because the department is a well defined unit which consists of a range of professional providers and which provides many different services.

The two phases to the modelling process are carried out separately and then both models are joined together. It is very important that the whole department is involved in this process so that consensus is obtained over the identification and ownership of the services being provided and consumed. However if this is not possible the most important criterion is that a person from each professional group is represented in the modelling phase.

Several small, interactive, multidisciplinary group training sessions were carried out with the departmental staff. In these sessions the staff were introduced to the concept of customer supplier modelling and were given specifically designed forms to list their different suppliers, customers and service or product provision. They were given one week to complete these forms and were encouraged to fill them in individually or by speciality. In the external modelling phase staff listed people, departments and outside organisations with whom the department worked with or relied upon. These groupings were categorised as either supplier, customer or both. A short, simple description of the product or service was given and a person or group of people were identified as the initiator or link person in the customer supplier relationship. After having defined the different relationships a preliminary model can be constructed. This is a formal depiction of all the different suppliers and customers, showing the service and product provision and their relationship to the department. This model was then taken back to the department to allow staff to comment and to make the necessary adjustments. The internal modelling phase follows a very similar process. After having defined the different internal relationships a formal model of the internal functioning of the department can be constructed.

ADVANTAGES AND PRACTICAL ISSUES

By constructing customer supplier models at a departmental level, staff are helped in developing a more formal understanding of how they integrate their work together internally and also how the department as a whole adapts externally to other hospital departments and outside organisations. This provides the framework for pin-pointing where current quality problems exist and for identifying weak inter-departmental and external relationships. This modelling technique aids interdisciplinary audit rather than specific medical, nursing or paramedical audit since it is describing the total health care package that the patient receives. It also helps staff to prioritise needs and provide the much needed structure for interdisciplinary audit activities. When any organisational changes are made their impact on the department can be assessed by evaluating the effect any changes have on the different customer supplier relationships.

However, as with all modelling techniques it also has its drawbacks and limitations. These include getting the commitment from all staff, identifying different levels of interaction and regularly updating the model when organisational changes occur. Thus the advantages of adopting this technique include:

- providing a holistic, interdisciplinary approach
- providing a framework for interdisciplinary audit and other quality improvement activities
- helping to prioritise needs

- identifying current work practice
- pin-pointing quality and organisational problems
- highlighting poor relationships
- acknowledging outside organisations

Important practical issues that need to be addressed include:

- provision of sufficient time to ensure initial modelling stages are effective
- involvement of all staff
- the need to address the problem of identifying different levels of interaction
- provision for regularly updating the model to reflect organisational changes

CONCLUSIONS / FURTHER WORK

The need to increase quality, reduce costs, and meet the internal and external contractual demands made on provider health care units, presents huge challenges for this decade (Koch 1991). This interdisciplinary systems approach, based on the use of customer-supplier modelling allows for the different provider groups, both internal and external, to join together and bring greater coherency to audit and quality improvement activities. The modelling method focuses on the total health care package that the patient receives, because of this it is felt that the technique reflects the holism inherent in medical care today. Thus it can be concluded that the approach put forward in this paper provides the framework for interdisciplinary audit and quality improvement and also offers opportunities to improve the health care system. This technique can be used at individual, speciality, directorate and unit level and is applicable to all areas of health care.

Having a framework for quality improvement without outcome measures, good information systems or knowledge of the effectiveness of interventions can make audit an unrewarding and tedious activity (Moss 1992). The next phase of this project will be involved with developing tools and techniques for testing the effectiveness of different interventions, measuring clinical output and understanding its relationship to health outcome. Information systems play a vital role in the support of the overall organisation. Therefore it is very important that the provision of information technology is examined and used appropriately as a support tool for quality improvement activities.

REFERENCES

Department of Health (1989), *Working for Patients*, HMSO, London.

Doyle, V., Carson, E.R., Sönksen, P.H., Winder, E. (1992), 'Total Quality Management in the Health Sector', Chytil, M.K., Duru, G, van Eimeren, W, Flagle, Ch.D. (eds), *Health Systems - the Challenge of Change, Proceedings of the 5th International Conference on System Science in Health Care*, Omnipress Publisher, Prague, 131 - 134.

Koch, H. (19991), 'Obstacles to Total Quality Management in Health Care', *International Journal of Health Care Quality Assurance,* 4 (3), 30-1.

Lohr, K.N. (1990), *Medicare: A Strategy for Quality Assurance Volume I,* National Academy Press, Washington D.C.

Moss, F. (1992), 'Quality in health care', *Quality in Health Care,* 1 (1), 1-3.

Oakland J. (1989), Total Quality Management, *Proceedings of the 2nd International Conference,* IFS Publications, Bedford, 4 - 17.

Relman, A.S. (1988), 'Assessment and Accountability: the third revolution', *N Eng J Med,* 321, 1220-1222.

Schein, E.H. (1987), *Organizational Culture and Leadership,* Jossey-Bass Publishers, San Francisco, London.

Vuori, H. (1992), 'Quality assurance in Finland', *BMJ,* 304, 162-4.

12 Usability Testing and Performance Evaluation — Empirical Study and Analysis of a Clinical Information System

**DAVID S. SIMPSON[1], DEREK SIMPSON[1] &
W. A. CORBETT[2]**

[1]*University of Teeside*
[2]*Department of Surgery, Middlesbrough General Hospital*

INTRODUCTION

The effectiveness of human-computer interaction is determined by the usability of the computer application and its interface. If designed and developed incorrectly, it can severely restrict the ability of a user to use the system efficiently and productively (Meister 1984). Techniques for evaluating human-computer interaction are comprehensively documented (Gould 1988; Gould, Boies, et al 1991). However, they often vary in the level of sophistication employed, and the accuracy and reliability of the data produced can deviate.

The most basic form of evaluation is the informal approach (i.e. direct observation), whereby system activity is observed while the user performs tasks. This method can be useful for highlighting frequently occurring errors and to identify parts of the system that may require modification. It can also help test the robustness of the system and assist in locating areas of user criticism or preference. The more formal approach to evaluation involves carrying out controlled experiments in which the system is more accurately observed. Although direct observation was used as part of this evaluative study, the principal approach was that of the controlled experiment. This involved groups of users carrying out set tasks and completing a detailed computer-based checklist/questionnaire; thus enabling them to describe their experiences while using the system, and allowing them to express their views about what they had done and why.

Strategic Issues in Health Care Management. Edited by M. Malek, J. Rasquinha and P. Vacani
© 1993 John Wiley & Sons Ltd

THE SYSTEM

The ERICA (Endoscopy Reporting Interface for Clinical Audit) system is a graphics-based environment for the management of endoscopic findings information. It has been developed to aid clinicians and associated medical personnel, and to facilitate greater communication of clinical results. Using the created facilities, icons can be mapped against sketch data to create pictorial depictions of gathered endoscopic information. Graphical representations of medical images have their workable parameters established at creation time and are stored within a series of medically agreed lexicons. The system contains a sequence of internal options including logical area confinement, icon to sketch fixing, textual integration, region of interest notation, and sketch/icon painting. ERICA runs through the MSDOS computer operating system, is written in the high level programming language Turbo Pascal, and has been developed to be intuitive and friendly to use.

RATIONALE

Objectives of Evaluation

Validating system design and usability can be a time and resource consuming activity. However, as stated by Gould and Lewis, (1985: 534); 'user testing will happen anyway: if it is not done in the developer's lab, it will be done in the customer's office". Certainly, the evaluation process cannot be achieved overnight, and it should be noted that time and effort worthy of its importance are necessary. Moreover, the potential benefits of the process may far outweigh the actual overheads and can include:

- Reduced training expenditure.
- Reduced support expenditure.
- Reduced necessity for system modifications and revisions.
- Increased system usability and user satisfaction.
- Greater system acceptance and effectiveness.
- Greater utilisation of available resources.
- Greater awareness of the need for 'user-centred' design.

Traditionally, evaluation plans involve an understanding of evaluation types. These could be formative or summative, - a view of evaluation conceived by Scriven in 1967 who used it originally in the context of educational research. Applying the notion to the development of computer-based systems, formative evaluation is the monitoring of the process and products of system development and the collection of user feedback, whereas summative evaluation is an assessment of the overall usability, impact, and effectiveness of system performance.

While it should be noted that this evaluative study concentrated primarily on summative evaluation, it was necessary to remain aware of formative evaluation and to incorporate aspects of it as required. The need to use several methods of evaluation in combination becomes more apparent when noting the multi-faceted nature of an evaluative study. Accordingly, the process of evaluation for this study was divided into four main objectives:

- To assess the usability of the system.
- To assess the capabilities and impact of the design principles.
- To identify areas where strengths and weakness exist.
- To assess the capabilities and impact of the evaluation methodology.

Consequently, the study undertaken was not only an evaluation of the system and the design principles used in its development, but also of the evaluation mechanism itself.

Choosing the Method

Since a principal aim of the study was the collection of valid and timely data in a practical and cost-effective manner, various decisions regarding the collection of observational data were made. While emphasis was placed on summative evaluation, it was decided that certain formative components were to be incorporated into the process, since often the only distinction made between the evaluation types lies in the use of the derived information (Hewett 1986).

Data Collection Methods

Usability criteria should be specified in a manner that makes them not only measurable but verifiable as well. However, certain usability criteria cannot be easily formulated in pure quantitative terms and communication problems can occur. This places an emphasis on the development of an evaluation plan that facilitates the collection of both objective and subjective data. To this end, it was decided to integrate the following approaches in the collection of evaluation data:

- Evaluation Checklist/Questionnaire
- Direct Observation
- User Comments

EVALUATION GROUPS

The importance of end-user evaluation is well documented (Mumford 1983; Brooke, 1986) and discussed in terms of human factors by Kruesi (1983), and Moreland, (1983). However, the degree to which end-user participation within the evaluation process is possible often depends on variables beyond the control of the system designer or developer. Several factors inhibited the use of actual end-users (i.e. clinicians) in this evaluative study: these included time constraints placed on the research project and end-users (i.e. scheduling difficulties and a shortage of access time); the physical impracticality of involving clinicians in the evaluation exercises; and, ultimately, a shortage of suitable and available end-users. Nevertheless, it was felt that the evaluative study was sufficiently flexible in its design and overall nature to enable a variety of personnel to take an active role in the exercise without compromising the validity and richness of the evaluation data.

Given the decision to carry out the primary study without actual clinicians, it was felt necessary to seek a reasonably large number of participants (i.e. evaluators). The question of sample size is often answered in the abstract based on statistical significance, however, because of differences in circumstances and goals, there is no definitive answer to the problem. In this instance, a minimal figure of around forty was established as the target amount because it was felt that this would provide a manageable number of participants and generate a considerable amount of data. This figure proved to be easy to obtain and helped to ensure the collection of a more than satisfactory amount of evaluation data.

The target population for the evaluative study - students, was identified early in the process.   The decision was taken to use three discrete groups of students (graduates and undergraduates) in the role of evaluators. - These students were from the School of Computing and Mathematics at the University of Teesside. To ensure an objective and balanced viewpoint, evaluators with a broad range of backgrounds and a wide spectrum of experience (i.e. technical and non-technical) were chosen. Each target group of students was approached, informed about the nature and objectives of the evaluation exercises, and given the opportunity to take part.

Following this initial contact, a significant number of volunteers emerged, and details of the final evaluation groups are supplied below:

- B.Sc. 1 Computer Science: Forty-four first year students with a varying mix of age and experience. Many recently attending school/college and having little practical experience in the use of computer-based information systems.
- B.Sc. 4 Computer Science: Twenty-two fourth year computer science students with an above average knowledge of the technical aspects of computer systems.
- M.Sc. Information Technology: Twenty students on an undergraduate conversion course providing, primarily, non-computer literate personnel with a variety of backgrounds.

Thus the evaluation groups were relatively widespread regarding the variables sex, age, education and background, and a range of different behavioural and attitudinal user reactions and responses were anticipated.

METHODOLOGY FOR EVALUATION

Characteristics of Users

To develop a user acceptable system it is important to clearly understand the specific user characteristics and to base system development around this information. The first step in the process is to carry out an assessment of the specific user characteristics. In the case of this particular study, the specific user characteristics of clinicians have been defined as:

- Intelligent.
- Computer naive.
- Little time to learn.
- Slightly irregular usage.
- Some computer antipathy.
- Little knowledge of system model.

The first of these characteristics is logical because of the very nature of the system's proposed user. The next places an onus on the system to ensure that the user is always given a reasonable idea of what the capabilities of the system are, and what is expected from them. By virtue of the users' profession, the third characteristic is true and suggests that the user has little, if any, time to acquire additional skills. This places an emphasis on the system to provide sufficient information for the user to carry out useful dialogue at all times. Furthermore, the user can be characterised as slightly irregular in terms of usage because individual clinicians do not, in general, carry out precisely the same procedure each day.

Whilst most clinicians view the introduction of information technology in the guise of microcomputers as useful for certain medical personnel, some still view them negatively and reject their use. This attitude strongly indicates a level of antipathy towards the technology. The final characteristic is derived because the user has little previous knowledge of the logical system model despite having an understanding of the intrinsic data properties involved.

As part of the evaluation process, it should be possible to relate the attributes of the final product back to the originally derived user characteristics. Clearly, both the features 'little time to learn' and 'slightly irregular usage' require the development of a self-explanatory system. Having established this fact, the attributes 'intelligent' and 'computer naive' reflect the level and type of system explanation required. Messages should be developed based on the assumption that the user is 'intelligent' but noting that little knowledge of computing or its inherent terminology is indicated. This point is also particularly relevant to the distinction 'some computer antipathy'. The final characteristic 'little knowledge of system model' defines the creation of a suitable model of the working process. The model should be developed to simulate current systems of work and provide clearly definable advantages. Users must be made at one with the system, and where practical the interface should relate to all derivation requirements.

System Usability Principles

Following the analysis of the specific user characteristics, the derived information is expanded to create a series of system usability principles (Smith and Mosier 198)]:

- Keep the dialogue simple and natural:

System dialogue should be free from irrelevant or rarely needed information, and it should appear in a natural and logical sequence.
- Speak the language of the users:
  Where possible all dialogue should be expressed in user familiar terms. Areas where any misunderstandings or misinterpretations are possible should always be avoided.
- Minimise the memory load of the users:
  System instructions should be clearly visible, easily retrievable, and informative.
- Remain consistent at all times:
  Users should be confident that the operational style of the system and all its inherent terminology is consistent throughout.
- Remain compatible:
  User conventions and expectations should be maintained wherever possible.
- Provide adequate, timely and appropriate feedback:
  Users should be given necessary feedback as and when required, and it should be made available within a reasonable period of time.
- Provide clearly marked paths:
  Explicit and easily accessed paths through the system should be made available. Information should be at hand to inform users where they are and what actions should be taken.
- Offer clearly marked exits:
  Clearly defined and easily accessed exit procedures should be provided.
- Provide system shortcuts wherever possible:
  Shortcuts should be designed to allow the system to cater for both novice and experienced users alike. Experienced users should be offered system shortcuts to increase productivity and to aid interaction.
- Offer appropriate, consistent and informative help:
  Help information should be explicit, easily accessed, and offer relevant assistance.
- Use good and informative error messages:
  Error messages should be expressed in clear and precise terms. They should indicate the problem and offer a solution wherever possible.
- Prevent errors wherever possible:
  Careful design and analysis can assist in minimising the possibility of errors occurring in the first place. Any potential errors should always be avoided.

Criterion-Based Approach to Evaluation

Substantial work has been carried out in an attempt to establish a series of guidelines for the design and development of computer-based systems (Smith and Mosier 1986; Gardner and Christie 1987). Despite the fact that these guidelines tend to vary in the degree of detail and content, the overall principles, or criteria, remain similar and are compatible. However, guidelines rarely consider the subjective needs and requirements of computer-based systems; as such they have limited use as a mechanism of evaluating their effectiveness. Therefore, a suitable evaluation metric must be established to allow those evaluating the system, 'the evaluators', to determine its overall usability. The information derived from the usability design process (i.e. system usability pri-based' approach to system evaluation and usability testing (Ravden and Johnson 1989).

The criterion-based approach is a practical tool, in the form of a checklist/questionnaire, which uses established design guidelines to provide a structured and systematic evaluation mechanism. It consists of a series of system specific questions based on ergonomics criteria or goals. These questions are designed to assess the usability of the system undergoing the evaluation process. The methodology enables an appraisal of the system by a variety of people, who can range in background and level of experience, and by representative users who may use the system in actual practice. The process can help to reveal:

- Any problem areas, difficulties or weaknesses.
- Areas that require improvement.
- The success or failure of the system
- Any positive aspects the system may exhibit.
- How successful the application is in meeting the stated criterion.

A key feature of the criterion-based approach is that evaluators must use the system undergoing evaluation to carry out a series of realistic tasks. These tasks should be designed as part of the evaluation process and should be representative of the work to be carried out by the system. They should test as much of the system and as many of its functions as possible. The tasks must be developed with great care and are crucial to the validity of the overall process of evaluation. The methodology can be used to assess design decisions and to test for usability both during and after system design and development. The specific evaluation criteria are placed under the following headings:

- Visual Clarity:
  The screen display of information should be explicit, well-organised, unambiguous and easy to read.
- Consistency:
  The appearance and operational technique of the system should be consistent at all times.
- Compatibility:
  The design and structure of the system should meet user conventions and expectations.
- Informative Feedback:
  Users should receive explicit, informative feedback on where they are, what actions are to be taken, and whether actions were successful or not.
- Explicitness:

The system's overall structure and mechanism of work should be clearly defined and set out.

- Appropriate Functionality:
  The system should address all user needs and requirements when carrying out tasks.
- Flexibility and Control:
  The style, design and facilities of the system should be sufficiently structured, flexible, and clear, to suit the user and leave them feeling in control.
- Error Prevention and Correction:
  The system should be designed to minimise the possibility of errors. Facilities should be available to detect and easily handle any errors that do occur.
- User Guidance and Support:
  Informative, easy to use and relevant assistance should be available both on and off the screen to assist the user to clearly understand the system.

To complement the checklist/questionnaire, a further criterion - General System Usability - is added. This section can facilitate the inclusion of a wider range of questions primarily related to the usability of the system in general terms.

Completing the Checklist/Questionnaire

Each of the individual sections is based on a different criterion or goal by which the system is measured. The specific criterion is described at the start of each section and consists of a heading, followed by a statement. A number of criterion specific questions (i.e. individual criteria) then follow. These questions are designed to assess whether the system meets the stated criterion and are not in any particular order of importance. To the right of each question are five columns labelled: 'No Answer', 'Always', 'Often', 'Occasionally' and 'Never'. Of these, 'Always' is the most favourable, whereas 'Never' is the least favourable.

Each question is 'marked' to indicate which best describes the evaluator's answer to the inquiry. Space is made available at the end of each section for comments to be added if required. This approach enables the evaluators to mention any aspects of the system, any problems, or any other considerations relevant to the criterion, which may have been omitted or not covered within the checklist/questionnaire.

Each section concludes with a criterion rating scale ranging from 'Very Satisfactory' to 'Very Unsatisfactory', 'Mainly Satisfactory' to 'Mainly Unsatisfactory', and 'No Answer' to 'Neutral'. This is designed to allow the evaluator the opportunity to provide a general assessment of the system in terms of the specific criterion and the questions within the section. The process concludes by asking a series of general system usability questions. On completion, each checklist/questionnaire can be summarised and compared for analytical purposes. This can help to reveal any confusion, misunderstandings, misinterpretations, and any contrasting aspects of usability.

TASK DESIGN AND CONSTRUCTION

Given the objectives of the evaluative study, it was decided to integrate several discrete system-based tasks and allow the evaluators to carry them out in a manner appropriate to the exercise. Using this particular approach, each of the tasks could be enlarged in its complexity and users could progress at their own speed. The tasks used in the study were formulated to contain all those aspects of the system normally employed when it is undergoing actual operation. They were designed to be an accurate representation of system-based tasks and to appear as realistic as possible. Each was capable of completion by the majority of evaluators, and each was created to examine the functionality of the system and its interface.

The final stage in the process was the construction of instructional material explaining the tasks to be carried out. This documentation was designed to be clear and leave evaluators in no doubt as to what they were required to do. It detailed a series of logical steps to be taken and highlighted the anticipated outcome for each stage. Furthermore, additional material provided to evaluators detailed the reason the exercise was taking place, offered a brief explanation of what the system is, who is to use it, and why it is being evaluated. This documentation included a brief rationale about the choice of evaluators, and how the participants could contribute and benefit the overall system design and development process. Moreover, the material explained how feedback was to play an important part in any future decisions, and that it was the system being tested, and not the individual.

CARRYING OUT THE EXPERIMENT

Eighty-six people took part in the controlled experiment and all successfully completed the evaluation exercise. Three sessions of evaluation were carried out - each dealing with a specific user group, and each staggered into blocks of forty minutes to allow uninterrupted access to the system. Before commencement of each exercise the individual evaluators were given a handbook of instructional material and asked to familiarise themselves with its contents for approximately one minute. Each of the handbooks contained a comprehensive step-by-step guide to using the system and each detailed a series of system specific tasks to be carried out by the user. On conclusion of the series of tasks (approximately twenty-five minutes), each user was given a copy of a completed ERICA graphic (i.e. a patient history) and asked to spend around five minutes attempting to replicate the document based on their recently acquired knowledge of the system

The primary goal of this evaluation process was threefold: first, to demonstrate the usability of the system and to enable the user to be exposed to as many aspects of it as reasonably possible; second, to ascertain if, after receiving a minimal amount of training, the user could successfully achieve a positive outcome using only the system undergoing evaluation; third, to facilitate an objective user opinion of the system after completing the pre-defined series of realistic, system-based tasks.

During each of the sessions, the evaluators were encouraged to question the actions of the system openly (i.e. think-aloud), and direct observation of all user behaviour was carried out. Important information is often obtained by merely observing the performance of users while carrying out tasks (Wright and Monk 1991). Immediate user difficulties while interacting with the system can identify confusions, common mistakes, logic errors, and misinterpretations. This approach was carried out to aid the study and helped to highlight some lack of interaction and areas where basic misunderstandings between the system and the user had occurred.

Furthermore, users were asked to spontaneously record any comments while interacting with the system, this information to be used by the user as an aide-memoire while completing the checklist/questionnaire if required. Immediately following the exercise, each user was asked to complete the on-line, computer-driven evaluation checklist/questionnaire. This style of user response data collection was adopted because it was felt that an on-line checklist/questionnaire has an advantage over the conventional paper-based system in terms of response time and reliability of data.

DATA ANALYSIS SUMMATION

Analysis of the evaluative study data generated a substantial amount of data and this is extensively discussed elsewhere. However, it is impractical to include this analysis within this document, therefore, this section looks in detail at the derived data in its aggregate form (see table 1). Here the overall user response figures for criterion one to nine, the system user rating of criterion one to ten, and the user experience values are each summed and examined. This analysis takes the form of an overall discussion, an individual group breakdown, and also looks at the positive grouped response of each criterion after the 'No Answer' values have been omitted.

Table 1.

Overall grand ratings total (criterion 1 to 9 inclusive)					
No Answer	Always	Often	Occasionally	Never	KEY
1002	4057	3135	785	137	Total
10.99	44.5	34.39	8.61	1.5	% Ratings (9116)

GRAND OVERALL, HOW DO YOU RATE THE SYSTEM IN TERMS OF CRITERION X? TOTAL (1 to 10 inclusive)						
No Answer	Very Satisfactory	Mainly Satisfactory	Neutral	Mainly Unsatisfactory	Very Unsatisfactory	KEY
55	249	429	111	16	0	Total
6.4	28.95	49.88	12.91	1.86	0.0	% Overall (860)

The overall summed data shows a positive grouped reaction to the system under evaluation of 78.89% and a user rating of 78.83%. The former value was weighted towards the 'Always' response (44.5%), whereas the latter moved towards 'Mainly Satisfactory' (49.88%). Analysis also shows that of a possible 9116 responses, there were 1002 (10.99%) 'No Answer' values and only 137 (1.5%) negative 'Never' replies. Moreover, the negative grouped response of 10.07% (918) was significantly less than the positive grouped reaction of 78.89% (7162). Discarding the 'No Answer' values further emphasises the positive aspects of the grouped figures; increasing the criterion response figure to 88.63% and the system user rating to 84.22%.

Looking closely at the system user rating category (see figure 1), the overall trend is extremely similar: the response pattern for all but one criterion moving from 'Mainly Satisfactory' to 'Very Satisfactory', then from 'Neutral' to 'Mainly Unsatisfactory'. Only Informative Feedback deviated from the pattern, moving from 'Mainly Satisfactory' (53.49%) to 'Neutral' (20.93%). The criterion Appropriate Functionality received the highest positive response (58.14%), whereas Error Prevention and Correction, and User Guidance and Support both recorded the lowest positive reaction (43.02%).

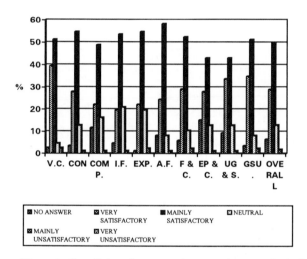

Figure 1. Overall, how do you rate the system in terms of criterion x?

Further analysis shows that, paradoxically, the criterion Visual Clarity had both the highest 'Very Satisfactory' (39.5%) and 'Mainly Unsatisfactory' (2.5%) responses. Furthermore, seven of the ten overall criterion recorded a 'Mainly Satisfactory' rating of 50.0% or more, only one received a 'Very Satisfactory' rating of less than 20.0% (Informative Feedback), and no 'Very Unsatisfactory' responses were recorded at all.

Taking the evaluation groups separately (see table 7.2 and figure 7.3), BSc 1 with a positive 81.17% criterion figure and a 79.32% system user rating, BSc 4 with a positive 74.36% criterion figure and a 75.0% system user rating, and MSc IT with a positive 78.87% criterion figure and an 82.0% system user rating, aligned closely with the grouped figures. The grouped negative 'Never' response of 137 (1.5%) was well distributed among the three data series: BSc 1 1.8%, BSc 4 1.03% and MSc IT 1.37%; whereas the 'No Answer' figure of 1002 (10.99%) was far more conclusively dispersed: BSc 1 9.01% (420 of 4664), BSc 4 16.12% (376 of 2332) and MSc IT 9.72% (206 of 2120). Each group is placed within the positive 80.0% plus range if the individual 'No Answer' values are discarded: BSc 1 84.81% and 84.29%, BSc 4 88.65% and 80.69%, and MSc IT 87.35% and 86.77%.

Table 2.

GRAND RATINGS TOTAL (criterion 1 to 9 inclusive)					
No Answer	Always	Often	Occasionally	Never	KEY
420	2257	1529	334	84	BSc 1 Total
9.01	48.39	32.78	7.16	1.8	% Ratings (4664)
376	861	873	198	24	BSc 4 Total
16.12	36.92	37.44	8.49	1.03	% Ratings (2332)
206	939	733	213	29	MSc IT Total
9.72	44.29	34.58	10.05	1.37	% Ratings (2120)

GRAND OVERALL, HOW DO YOU RATE THE SYSTEM IN TERMS OF CRITERION X? TOTAL (1 to 10 inclusive)						
No Answer	Very Satisfactory	Mainly Satisfactory	Neutral	Mainly Unsatisfactory	Very Unsatisfactory	KEY
26	137	212	55	10	0	BSc 1 Total
5.91	31.14	48.18	12.5	2.27	0.0	% Overall (440)
18	52	113	34	3	0	BSc 4 Total
8.18	23.64	51.36	15.45	1.36	0.0	% Overall (220)
11	60	104	22	3	0	MSc IT Total
5.5	30	52	11	1.5	0.0	% Overall (200)

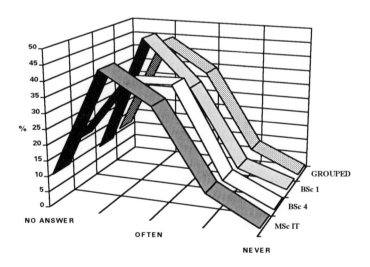

Figure 2. All Criterion Rating Chart

Analysis of the positive grouped responses (see figure 3), after discarding the 'No Answer' values, shows the positive aspects of each specific criterion to be extremely encouraging. No criterion recorded a grouped figure of less than 84.29%, and the highest positive reaction was a significant 96.42%. Furthermore, four of the criterion under evaluation received a positive grouped response of over 90.0%, and a summation of the aggregate data shows an overall positive grouped figure of 89.18%.

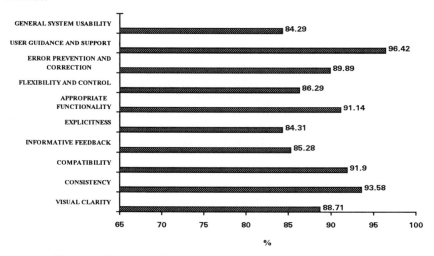

Figure 3. Criterion positive grouped response chartCriterion psitive grouped responses (minus 'no answer' values)

CONCLUSIONS

A computer-based information system has the parallel responsibilities of guiding and controlling user actions according to common requirements, and of assisting the user to fulfil tasks as easily and speedily as possible. This evaluative study has been carried out in an attempt to compare system characteristics with a set of pre-established criteria (each located within the specific criterion), and to determine the degree of correspondence to each. The study has generated a substantial amount of data, and analysis has identified several areas where usability problems occur - for example deficiencies in system flexibility and functionality, and basic omissions within certain system-driven facilities. Furthermore, the data also indicates some variation in user expectations and demands, despite the user groups being largely homogeneous in terms of behaviour and evaluative tasks. However, the data also includes a considerable number of positive responses for every criterion. The ubiquitous nature of this user reaction is significant and as such is strongly supportive of the work carried out during the design, development and implementation of the system.

Throughout this evaluative study several different forms of user testing and system evaluation have been used. Most concentrated on the ability or inability of the user to perform a series of tasks using the system undergoing evaluation. Set tasks, direct observation, user comments, and a checklist/questionnaire were employed to collect data from users. An empirical measurement technique, derived and adapted from the criterion-based approach to system evaluation, was then used to analyse the material and to carry out a detailed assessment of the system. This approach generated a considerable amount of information, and the conclusions of the analysis are succinctly presented and discussed (also see data summation). Moreover, the study helped to formulate a number of empirically motivated points regarding the usability of the system and the usefulness of the evaluation methodology.

Usability

The results obtained from the evaluative study strongly suggest that a high level of system usability has been achieved. Furthermore, there is little, if any, evidence to say that any of the adopted design principles are incorrect. This has led to the formulation of a number of empirically derived points regarding the usability of the system and the correctness of the design principles:

- User performance objectives must be established as part of the initial product definition.
- The design principles can increase system usability, and are applicable and exportable to various situations.
- The importance of remaining aware of cognitive science and human factors during each stage of the design and development process should not be minimised.
- It is necessary to focus on the needs of users and to involve them actively in each iteration of design and development.
- There must be a willingness to design decision changes based on user comments and response. Good systems can only be created by following an iterative design and development process.
- Increased usability often runs parallel with increased creation effort (i.e. the more usability, the more resources required) - this result concurs with several reports, notably Myers (1988). However, the potential benefits are large and can include: easier learning, cost effectiveness, better user acceptance, reduced error rates, and improved throughput.

Additional evidence regarding the usability of the system is provided when considering the supposition put forward previously That is, after receiving only a minimal amount of system training, the user should be able to achieve a positive outcome with relative ease. To test this, after completing a series of set tasks, each user was given a completed ERICA graphic (i.e. a patient history) and asked to spend around five minutes attempting to replicate the document. In each instance, the user successfully completed the task, thus confirming that, provided users are aware of the task to be performed and know how to map it to the system, the usability built into the system can facilitate positive user-system interaction.

In summary, the analysis has identified certain usability problems, some basic omissions, and a slight variation in user expectation and demand. However, the negative aspects of the derived information were minimal. On the other hand, the number of positive responses accrued throughout the study was significant. This affirms that users were positively supportive of both:

- The work carried out to build usability into the system.
- The research and development of the utilised design principles.

Evaluation Methodology

The evaluation methodology used within this study involved adapting key principles put forward by Gould and Lewis (1985), on usability design (i.e. early focus on users and tasks, empirical measurement, and iterative design and development), and mapping them to the criterion-based approach to system evaluation. This process required a clear understanding of specific user characteristics and the formulation of a suitable evaluation metric. Furthermore, it involved measuring system development and usability against user-led criteria, and an iterative series of questioning, observation, and analysis.

Detailed analysis of the evaluation methodology helped to highlight several important points regarding system evaluation, usability testing, and this particular approach to evaluation:

- Reliable and rich data can be gathered in a manner that is both practical and time efficient.
- Empirical data is vital to the process of evaluation to ensure that accurate and informative information is derived.
- Computer-based information systems of quality can only be generated by testing with users and being prepared to modify design decisions based on their responses. Clearly, ease of use can only be evaluated through use.
- A range of measures, subjective and objective, is important to test if usability goals are achieved.
- The richness of information derived from just talking and listening to users should not be underestimated.
- Summative and formative evaluation must be integrated into the procedure according to the stage in the evaluation-design process and the evaluation issues present. This requires the designers/developers making early decisions regarding the goals of the system, the goals of the design process, the goals of the evaluation process, and the benchmarks by which to assess the achievement of these goals.
- The overall nature and flexibility of design embodied in the evaluation methodology facilitates the collection of valid, high quality data, without the necessity to involve actual end-users (i.e. representative users) in the evaluation process.

- The evaluation methodology can be modified to suit the product, time available, and the users. For example, the number of questions used within the checklist/questionnaire can be varied and may be reduced if required, but only with great care. In the case of this evaluative study, given the large number of positive responses recorded, the fundamental outcome would remain the same despite a reduction in the number of questions used. However, where a more widespread user reaction was recorded, a reduction in the amount of questions would make the isolation of specific factors more problematic.

To summarise, through use of this evaluation methodology, a substantial amount of user feedback was obtained and analysed without the requirement to deploy cumbersome or unnecessarily rigid methods of evaluation. Moreover, unlike the experimental testing approach to system evaluation and usability testing, this technique proved to be cost-effective and adaptable, provided an abundance of high quality data, and contributed to bringing the needs of the user and the designer/developer closer together.

REFERENCES:

Brooke J B, (Sept 1986), 'Usability engineering in office product development', Harrison M D and Monk A F. (eds), *People and Computers,* Proceedings of the Second Conference of the British Computer Society HCI Specialist Group, Cambridge University Press.

Gardner M M, Christie B, (1987), *Applying cognitive psychology to user interface design,* John Wiley and Sons Press.

Gould J D, (1988), 'How to design usable systems', Helander. (ed), *Handbook of Human-Computer Interaction,* 757/789.

Gould J D, Boies S J, et al, (Jan. 1991), 'Making usable, useful, productivity-enhancing computer applications', *Communications of the Association for Computing Machinery (ACM),* 34, 74/86.

Gould J D, and Lewis C H, (1985), 'Designing for usability: key principles and what designers think', *Communications of the Association for Computing Machinery (ACM),* 28, 300/311

Hewett T T, (Sept 1986), 'The role of iterative evaluation in designing systems for usability', Harrison M D and Monk A F. (eds), *People and Computers,* Proceedings of the Second Conference of the British Computer Society HCI Specialist Group, Cambridge University Press.

Kruesi E, (1983), 'The human engineering task area', *IEEE Computer,* 16:11, 86/93.

Meister D, (1984), 'A catalogue of ergonomic design methods', *Proceedings of the 1984 International Conference on Occupational Ergonomics,* 2, 17/25.

Moreland D V, (1983), 'Human factors for terminal interface design', *Communications for the Association of Computing Machinery (ACM),* 26:7, 484/493.

Mumford E, (1983), 'Designing participatively', *Manchester Business School Publication*, UK.

Myers B A, (1988), 'Creating user interfaces by demonstration', *Perspectives in Computing*, Academic Press Inc., 22.

Ravden S, Johnson G, (1989), 'Evaluating usability of human-computer interfaces', *Ellis Horwood Books on Information Technology*.

Scriven M, (1967), 'The methodology for evaluation', Tyler R U, Ragne R M and Scriven M. (eds.), *Perspectives on Curriculum Education*, Chicago: Rand McNally.

Smith S L, Mosier J, (1986), 'Guidelines for designing user-interface software', *The Mitre Corporation*, Bedford, Massachusetts, USA, Report Number: MTR-10090. (ADA177198).

Wright P, Monk A F, (1991), 'A cost-effective method for use by designers', *International Journal of Man-Machine Studies*, 35, 891/912.

13 The Use of an Issue-Information Matrix in the Rapid Evaluation of Health Services Performance

STANISLAW ORZESZYNA, MICHEL C. THURIAUX & STEPHEN A. SAPIRIE

World Health Organisation, Switzerland

INTRODUCTION

Rapid evaluation method (REM) is a method which aims at identifying operational problems in order to take managerial action, through brief sample surveys carried out in health care facilities and the community. It has been used to assess the performance and quality of health services in six countries (Botswana, China, Madagascar, Papua New Guinea, Uganda, Zambia) between 1988 and 1992. This paper describes the use of one component of REM, *viz.*, the issue-information matrix, in the preparation and design of rapid evaluations.

BACKGROUND

Managing health services requires relevant and timely information on the performance of health care institutions and staff and on the health status of the population. Most health services require health personnel to record extensive routine data on many forms, and to forward these to higher levels of the system. This overburdens health staff and contributes to a vicious circle of underutilization and poor data quality; the data are furthermore often criticized for being unreliable and are rarely analysed nor used for management purposes.

There is thus a need for methods which accurately, quickly and economically produce the information necessary for decision making. Methods of rapid assessment of performance in health care have recently been described by Bryce *et al.* (1992) and by Anker *et al.* (1993). REM is designed on the premise that health service managers are already familiar with basic service statistics but need more information on the quality of care given and the degree of client satisfaction and response. It entails the participation of national programme managers and staff in the design and implementation of the evaluation in a relatively short period of time.

Strategic Issues in Health Care Management. Edited by M. Malek, J. Rasquinha and P. Vacani
© 1993 John Wiley & Sons Ltd

The initial step in REM is for national authorities to state the uses to which the results of the evaluation will be put, and to identify those programmes and services likely to be involved, as well as to decide on the topics and issues to be included, and those to be excluded. This step is taken by high-level decision makers, usually senior officials of the ministry of health. Having decided on these aspects, national authorities appoint a "core group" to take responsibility for the design and implementation of REM. This includes confirming the main issues the REM will address (keeping in mind the use to be made of the resulting information), specifying the types of information to be collected, identifying possible sources for this information, setting the schedule for producing the results, and making the necessary logistical arrangements, including staff, transport, and budgetary matters.

DEVELOPING THE ISSUE-INFORMATION MATRIX

Designing an issue-information matrix is an important early step in the preparation of a REM. The matrix follows a logical process for identifying relevant information on the basis of selected health problems and those aspects of health care delivery which are by decision-makers to deserve review. This process, which enables the core group to identify appropriate information sources and methods, is presented on Figure 1.

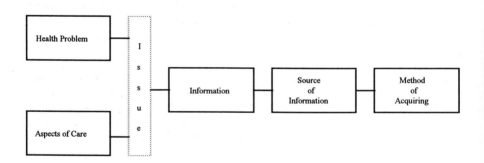

Figure 1: Identifying relevant information

A complete matrix designed in one of the countries is shown in Annex 1. A matrix may contain considerable detail, and experience shows that the process of creating it proves very useful in identifying those aspects of the service to be assessed and the information needed to make the assessment.

We shall proceed, step by step, with the description of how such a matrix is used. Health problems are listed vertically in the leftmost column, and the major aspects of health care delivery are placed in the two top rows of the matrix. There are, therefore, two ways to recognize an important "issue" to be addressed during REM -

either by defining a health problem, or by recognizing an important aspect of health care delivery.

The first step is to define the major health and health care delivery problems to be addressed. Figure 2 presents some major health problems which were defined in one of the REMs. Usually, within a broad health subject, a number of more detailed and specific problems are identified. In one country, for example, a major health subject was maternal health, within which the group chose obstructed labour, hypertension and anaemia as problems deserving in-depth study. Additional health problems chosen were AIDS and child nutrition and could similarly be subdivided.

Health Problem
Maternal Health - Obstructed labour - hypertension - anaemia
AIDS
Nutrition

Figure 2: Major health problems defined in a REM

Figure 3 presents an example of important health care delivery aspects identified in a REM. These aspects include community involvement (client knowledge, attitudes, practices, satisfaction and participation), technical performance (staff knowledge, attitudes, skills and satisfaction and adherence to standard procedures), management (including planning, use of information and supervision), training, and resources.

Community involvement		Technical performance		Management			T r a i n i n g	R e s o u r c e s
Staff knowledge Attitudes Skills Satisfaction	Participation	Knowledge Attitudes Practices	Staff procedures	Planning Administration	Information	Supervision		

Figure 3: Major aspects of health services delivery

As previously mentioned, the task of building the matrix starts from either of two dimensions — a health problem or a health delivery aspect. The identification of these two elements leads to the identification of the relevant issues and the corresponding information needs, which are placed in the matrix at the intersection of the appropriate row and column. An example of this is given in Table 1. In this case, the working group decided that an important health problem in the country was unsatisfactory maternal health, and in particular, deaths due to obstructed labour. At the same time, the group suspected a low level of technical performance of staff in terms of their knowledge and skills in identifying risk factors related to obstructed labour. The crucial step was to specify relevant information items at the cross sections of the two dimensions just described (knowledge of risk factors and the referral experience). The group then made a list of possible sources of information which could be used to address the 'issue'. In this case these sources included staff interview (to assess staff knowledge and attitudes), exit interview (to find out what in fact was done during encounter), record check (to find out the extent and appropriateness of referrals).

Table 1. Building an issue-information matrix

	Technical Performance	
	Staff knowledge, attitudes skills, satisfaction	Staff procedures
Maternal health	Identifying risk factors	Referral of obstructed labour cases
- *Obstructed labour*	Source: health staff Method: staff interview	Source: health facility Method: record check
		Source: patients Method: exit interview

DATA COLLECTION INSTRUMENTS

The issue-information matrix provided the basis to develop survey instruments; in most countries these include:

• **Review of clinical records** — these determine whether procedures were recorded properly and in evaluating case management of certain 'tracer' conditions. For instance, in reviewing antenatal care, a checklist of those items (age, blood pressure, obstetric history), which should be recorded on a clinic record card indicates the extent to which those standard tasks were properly recorded (and therefore carried out). Specific items which were often missing were identified for further investigation. Handling of high risk cases can be monitored well through record checks.
• **Clinic exit interviews** — patients are interviewed immediately after consultation or contact with the health services, in order to assess the functioning of the health care facility from the point of view of the client. Questions include items on patient satisfaction or dissatisfaction with the services rendered, and other problems encountered in seeking health care. Exit interviews also give an

opportunity to determine if clinics are providing correct health education messages: asking women leaving the antenatal clinic to list some of the warning signs associated with pregnancy provided feedback on how well educational messages regarding these signs were understood by patients. Asking women whether specific procedures were carried out during the clinic session (blood pressure measurements, abdominal palpation, tetanus toxoid injection) also gave some indication of quality of antenatal care.

- **Health staff interviews** — these provide information from health workers about attitudes, issues pertaining to management and supervision, job satisfaction, education and training, as well as to identify perceived problems and list suggestions for improvements. Different questionnaires were applied for various categories of health staff.

- **Observation of task performance** — this is one of the most effective ways of learning what actually happens during the patient-staff encounter. Although the procedure is time-consuming and sometimes can influence performance, it was employed in several countries to supplement information on quality of care obtained from record reviews.

- **Community and staff focus group discussions** — these are in-depth discussions among a small group of individuals chosen from a specific target group under the guidance of a trained facilitator (Khan 1991). Focus group discussions are especially useful for eliciting information on feelings, attitudes and behaviour, or information about sensitive issues which cannot be easily obtained in a household interview. They are often used to provide information about community perceptions on issues related to health problems, to health care, and service performance and acceptability. Focus group discussions can also be conducted with health staff, including traditional birth attendants and public health nurses; providing better understanding of the work done by the staff, and the problems they perceive in carry out their tasks.

- **Checking facilities, equipment and supplies** — this includes checks of the physical structure of the facility, equipment, supplies, and other items the presence and good condition of which are important for the patients' needs and the quality of the type of care chosen for review. Both the availability of the items in the checklist and their condition (satisfactory or unsatisfactory) were observed and recorded.

- **Household interviews** — these provide a means of measuring the knowledge and practice of people who do not use the service, were carried out in two countries only, in the catchment areas of the health facilities selected for the REM.

Use of information for action

A fundamental principle of REM is the prompt application of acquired information in the process of managerial decision-making. Tables 2 and 3 show examples of how managerial issues and information collected in a REM were used in defining actions contemplated by decision-makers.

Table 2. Action regarding community awareness

Issue	Findings	Proposed Managerial Action
Community awareness of family planning	Misconceptions with regard to family planning; under-utilization of family planning services	To provide health education materials in clinics

Table 3. Action regarding health status performance

Issue	Findings	Proposed managerial action
Health staff performance with regards to lowering maternal mortality	Poor staff knowledge of maternal mortality cases and high risk factors	To provide technical guidelines to standardize the expected performance of health staff in the area of maternal health

DISCUSSION

The process of defining and using an issue-information matrix raises several issues. Namely:

- **Identification of health and health services problems; definition of data needs.** The importance of this phase of the exercise cannot be overemphasized. The participation of national health staff as diverse as ministry officials, physicians, midwives, training tutors, and nurses in charge of a health centre is an important asset to the meaningfulness of the process, but problem identification can be a lenghty process and usually takes several days to complete before a consensus is reached, although initial problem selection can usually be achieved in half a day.
- **Preparation of instruments.** Experience showed that the survey instruments were in many cases changed immediately prior to the actual field work. This may have an adverse effect on the quality of interviewing and data collection. It should be therefore emphasized that unless this is essential, the survey tools should not be changed, after they have been pre-tested, revised and approved by the core group.
- **Use of data to produce information.** The quantitative information produced by REM must be tabulated and analysed quickly. It is of primary importance that his information be presented to programme managers as early as feasible after the fieldwork. The range of this period of time in the 6 countries varied from a few days to several weeks. In most countries the results of REM were presented at a meeting with the participation of health authorities responsible for

MCH and served as a basis for policy recommendations. Developing meaningful issue-information matrices in an early stage of the REM should allow the amount of data to be limited to that really necessary in the few areas to be focussed on.

CONCLUSION

Rapid evaluation method is a useful tool to collect useful, relevant information and to present it quickly to decision makers in the form which is easy to understand. An essential step in this process is the definition of the issue information matrix. The matrix facilitates the logical flow of activities starting from agreeing on an important health problem within an issue area, defining the information sources and information collection methods. This method should be strengthened and improved in the forthcoming REM exercises.

REFERENCES

Anker, M., Guidotti, R.J., Orzeszyna, S., Sapirie, S.A., Thuriaux, M.C. (1993), 'Rapid evaluation methods (REM) of health services performance: methodological observations', *World Health Organization Bulletin*, 71 (1), 15-21.

Bryce, J., Toole, M.J., Waldman, R.J., Voigt, A. (1992), 'Assessing the quality of facility-based child survival services', *Health Policy and Planning*, 7 (2), 155-163.

Khan, E.M., Anker, M., Patel, B.C., Barge, S., Sadhwani, H., Kohle, R. (1991), 'The use of focus groups in social and behavioural research: some methodological issues', *World Health Statistics Quarterly*, 44, 145-149.

Annex 1 An actual issue-information matrix developed in one of the countries

Aspects of service	Community action		Technical performance		Management			Training	Resources
HEALTH PROBLEM	Community KAPS*	Participation	Staff KASS*	Staff procedure	Planning, administration	Information	Supervision		
ANTENATAL CARE	Attitude to referral; Knowledge of maternal deaths and high risk	Attitude toward ANC*	Knowledge of maternal deaths and high risk	Risk identification; Risk management; Administration of tetanus toxoid; Frequency of ANC* consultations RC OBS SQ EX	Antenatal target set	Coverage with ANC* care; Risk; Follow-up	Number of supervisory visits;	Adequacy of training; Understanding of job description; What to add to basic and post-basic training	Transport available; Budget for petrol; Availability of drugs and equipment
DELIVERY CARE		What can be done?	Deaths? Causes? Constraints; Attitude to hospital	Referrals RC SQ*	No. of village midwives registered RC SQ*	Delivery records maintained; Deaths registered; Referrals recorded; Quality of records	Number of supervisory visits; VBA* supervision SQ RC*	How much done for in-service VBA* training	Availability of equipment and IV sets, suction devices, ergometrine
POST-NATAL CARE	Information received		Satisfaction with performing tasks	FP* education and service; Number of PNC* RC SQ*	Immunization start; FP given; Check-up RC SQ*		Number of supervisory visits; VBA* supervision SQ RC		
FAMILY PLANNING Fertility, Low coverage, Supplies	Knowledge of available FP* services; Use of various methods of FP*		Knowledge of FP* targets; Satisfaction with FP* coverage; Knowledge of eligible women	No of clinics a week; The extent to which these clinics are advertized	FP* targets set	FP* records; Eligible couples recorded; FP* coverage calculated	Number of supervisory visits; VBA* supervision SQ RC*		Availability of educational materials & contraceptive supplies
IMMUNIZATION Tetanus toxoid Polio	Awareness of tetanus and polio; Clinic schedule; Use/non-use; Knowledge of schedules	Possible support; Participation, Drop-out	Coverage; Dropout; Acceptance of policy of few contraindications	Tetanus toxoid as part of ANC*; Education; Administration technique of immunization OBS EX*	Feedback received; Temperature of fridge recorded SQ RC OBS	Polio and TT coverage; Use of data to determine non-coverage; Dropout rate	Number of supervisory visits; VBA supervision SQ RC*		Availability of working fridge
DATA COLLECTION METHOD	FG	FG	SQ	Various	SQ RC OBS	RC SQ	SQ RC	SQ	OBS

* **Abbreviations:** ANC Antenatal care; EX Exit questionnaire; FG Focus group discussion; FP Family planning; IV Intravenous; KAPS Knowledge, attitudes, practices, satisfaction; KASS Knowledge, attitude, skills, satisfaction; OBS Observation of health facility; PNC Postnatal care; RC Record check; SQ Staff interview; TT Tetanus toxoid; VBA Village birth attendant

14 Acceptance and Diffusion of National Standards in General Practice

A. M. ZWAARD, J. DALHUYSEN, H. MOKKINK & R. GROL

Nijmegen University, The Netherlands

INTRODUCTION

Setting standards and criteria for medical care in general practice is crucially important for the quality of care (Donabedian 1986). In the Netherlands, the Dutch College of General Practitioners (Nederlands Huisartsen Genootschap) has attempted to set national standards and has been developing them since 1987. They are meant to reflect the 'state of art' in Dutch family practice and to be used as guidelines for medical audit, quality assurance, evaluation in vocational training and continuing medical education. The first national standard, non-insulin dependent Diabetes Mellitus, was published in January 1989 in the Dutch scientific journal for family doctors, which is the College magazine. About 60% of general practitioners receive the national standards in this way. Standards now are part of CME-activities and are being used in vocational training.

It is well known that compliance to guidelines for medical practice is poor (Frame et.al. 1984; Schreiner et.al. 1988; Ornstein et.al. 1989; Selinger et al 1989; Yoong et al 1992; Stange et al 1992). It is also known that simply developing and publishing standards is not enough to change practice behaviour. It is important to know attitudes of care providers towards the standards or concrete guidelines and to know what the reasons are for not working in accordance to these guidelines (Fishbein and Azjen 1975). These factors can give direction to an implementation strategy.

At the Centre for Quality Assurance Research in Family Practice of the Faculty of Family Medicine of Nijmegen University, research is carried out to evaluate different strategies for the implementation of standards and guidelines among Dutch general practitioners. In an experimental design with two regions, an experimental and a control region, strategies are being evaluated to disseminate and implement the standards in general practice.

Strategic Issues in Health Care Management. Edited by M. Malek, J. Rasquinha and P. Vacani
© 1993 John Wiley & Sons Ltd

As a part of this research a recent survey was carried out among Dutch general practitioners, and the survey results were compared with earlier surveys among general practitioners (Grol 1990). The questions in the survey sought responses about:

- Attitudes towards national standards and which developments are expected in future
- The ways in which general practitioners are informed about the guidelines in the different standards for medical practice
- The main factors preventing implementation of standards

METHOD

A questionnaire was sent to a randomised sample of 500 Dutch general practitioners. It was also sent to all the general practitioners practising in the two regions of the implementation study (the control and experimental regions). In total questionnaires were sent to 1628 general practitioners (from a total of approximately 6500). The questionnaire was sent 3 years after the publication of the first national standard. It contained a mixture of open and closed questions about how well informed the respondents were about the standard setting campaign, how well informed the respondents were about the existence of a number of concrete standards and in which way they were informed about the content of the different standards. The questionnaire also contained a number of 16 different guidelines, which are the key features of 6 different standards. The questions asked were if one was acquainted with the content of these guidelines, if one did agree with these guidelines and if one said to be working in accordance with these guidelines. The GP's were also asked to answer several questions on possible problems or reasons for not working according to the standards.

Doctor and practice characteristics assessed included: age, years of experience as a general practitioner, membership of the Dutch College (NHG), involvement in education or vocational training and degree of urbanisation of practice location.

After 4 weeks, a repeat questionnaire was sent to those who had not responded and where necessary, a reminder was sent after a further 4 weeks.

In order to trace selection bias, 80 doctors were randomly selected from the non-respondents. In telephone interviews a selection of the questions from the questionnaire was used.

RESULTS

The response rate was 67%. The age distribution of the respondents was almost the same as the distribution of the national population of family doctors, the respondents being slightly younger than the national population. Among the respondents 70% were members of the Dutch College, versus 61% of the national population.

The non-respondents proved to be less well informed about individual guidelines and agreed less with these guidelines.

ACCEPTANCE OF NATIONAL STANDARDS

Almost 90% of the respondents said they were well informed or very well informed about the national standard setting campaign, versus 77% in 1989. 68% of the respondents believed that national standards should not become obligatory. About the same percentage said that standards make the tasks of the family doctor clear for the community. 36% said standards can be abused by others, e.g. patients demanding things the doctor doesn't want to do, or insurance companies trying to control the course of action in future practice. 87% think standards are a professional responsibility for general practice. One is not very afraid the guidelines themselves will restrict daily work. It still remains the personal responsibility of each doctor to decide how to act in specific situations. 77% of the respondents consider that working in accordance to standards can make work more efficient and cost-effective.

Table 1. Attitudes to national standards

national standards:	*Strongly Agree* March 1989 (n=453)	*Strongly Agree* April 1992 (n=1069)
— should not become obligatory	56%	68%
— can be abused by others	23%	36%
— make the tasks of the family doctor clear to the community	61%	67%
— are restrictive for the doctor	20%	18%
— are professional responsibility of family doctors		87%
— should be obligatory in continuing education (CME)		60%
— are cost-effective		77%

ATTITUDES TO THE ROLE AND FUNCTION OF NATIONAL STANDARDS

Standards can play an important role in CME-activities. They are less fit for selective purposes (selection in vocational training and recertification). In vocational training (85%) and in peer review and medical audit (84%) the standards play an important role. They also have an important function in the discussions in GP-groups how to act in practice situations. 81% of the respondents said standards can play a role to establish a course of action in GP-groups.

Comparing these results with three years ago, many more doctors are informed about the national standard setting campaign and they see a bigger role of national standards for educational purposes than three years ago. The percentage of doctors that (strongly) agree that standards can be abused by others (patients, insurance companies, government) increased from 23% to 36% of the respondents, an increase of more than 50%.

Table 2. Attitudes to the usefulness of national standards

Usefulness of national standards:	Very good Sept. 1991 (n=399)	Very good April 1992 (n=1069)
— in CME-activities	84%	89%
— recertification/registration	39%	36%
— relection in vocational training	26%	23%
— education in vocational training	85%	—
— research purpose	66%	63%
— peer review and audit	84%	90%
— how to handle in GP-groups	81%	90%

KNOWING ABOUT SPECIFIC STANDARDS

A list of eight published standards were presented, asking if the GP was aware of the existence of these standards. One to two years after the publication of these standards almost all the respondents knew about most of them. Less than one year after publication of the standards on hypertension and cholesterol 93% of the respondents said they were aware about their existence.

The exact content of the term 'knowing about' is not clearly defined. It may mean 'have heard of it' or even 'know the precise content of the standard'.

Table 3. The way GP's were informed about standards (n=1069)

College magazine	89
Other medical journal	22
Informal contact with colleagues	57
CME-activities	45
Discussing in gp-groups	68
Lay-press coverage	3
Pharmaceutical representatives	17

THE WAY IN WHICH GP's WERE INFORMED

Doctors were asked how they were informed about the existence or the context of the standards. More than one answer was permitted. 89% said they were informed about individual standards by reading the College magazine. Although 61% of Dutch GPs are members of the College, and automatically subscribed to the magazine, there is probably a greater number of readers. Other medical journals in the Netherlands were mentioned as a source of information by 22% of the respondents. 68% of the respondents stated that conversation about the standards in their GP-group was how they were informed about the standards. Informal personal contact with colleagues (57%) and CME-activities (45%) were also important diffusion channels for information on standards. Pharmaceutical representatives (17%) and lay-press coverage (3%) were less important sources of information.

It seems that specific diffusion channels for general practitioners, such as the College magazine and GP-group activities are the most important for information about the standards. Also a combination of different channels seems to be of importance for the dissemination of information about standards among general practitioners.

Table 4. Being informed about the existence of concrete standards

	Month of publication in College Magazine	Knowing this standards exists (April 1992 (n=1069)
Acute medial otitis	June '90	94%
Sore throat	August '90	83%
Acne vulgaris	April '91	84%
Hypertension	August '91	93%
Chronic venous leg ulcer	June '91	71%
Cholesterol	Nov. '91	93%
Dementia	Dec '91	62%

KNOWING SPECIFIC GUIDELINES, AGREEING WITH THESE GUIDELINES AND WORKING IN ACCORDANCE TO THESE GUIDELINES

For 16 distinct guidelines (key features of 6 different national standards) GPs were asked if they were acquainted with them. If the GP was acquainted, they were then asked if they were working according to these guidelines. For two of the six national standards the results will be discussed.

Regarding hypertension, 97% of the respondents were acquainted with the guideline that at least three blood pressure measurements are necessary before a definite case of hypertension can be diagnosed. 90% agreed with this guideline with 87% stating they were following it. 92% were acquainted with the guideline that a diuretic or a beta-blocker are drugs of first choice in treating hypertension. 60% agreed and said they were following this guideline. A third guideline about hypertension says that if the patient is less than 30 old, a specialist referral is necessary. 77% were acquainted with this guideline, 67% agreed and 62% stated that they were working according to this guideline.

From the national standard for Non Insulin Dependent Diabetes Mellitus one of the key features, states that the fasting blood glucose level to be achieved is < 6.7 mmol/l. 91% were acquainted with this guideline, 81% agreed and 72% said they were following this guideline. A second guideline recommends that every three months the weight should be measured. 85% were acquainted with this guideline, 81% agreed and 62% said they were following this guideline. A third guideline deals with marking the patient records of diabetics. 84% were acquainted with this guideline, 78% agreed and 56% said they were following this guideline.

The conclusion is that different guidelines from national standards are well known. The number of respondents who agree differ for the different guidelines and the percentage of respondents working according to the guidelines show an even bigger variation.

Table 5. Knowing guidelines, agreeing with guidelines and working according to guidelines, (n=1069)

	Knowing the guideline	Agreeing with the guideline	Working according to the guideline
Standard hypertension			
3 measurements necessary	97%	90%	87%
Diuretic/beta-blocker drug first choice	92%	60%	60%
Less than 30 years old specialist referral	77%	67%	62%
Standard Diabetes Mellitus Type-II			
Fasting blood glucose level < 6.7 mmol/l	91%	81%	72%
Every 3 months weight control	84%	81%	62%
Marking the charts of diab.patients	84%	78%	56%

PROBLEMS WITH WORKING ACCORDING TO STANDARDS

A list of possible factors that could be reasons for not working according to standards was proposed. One of the major problems is changing the old routines. 39% said they fall back easily into old routines. 30% said that patients could present difficulties, requesting things the doctors didn't want to do. The same percentage said (different) medical specialist work can be a problem. The fact that every patient is different is a problem for 33% of the respondents. Working according to standards can cost extra time or money (29%), doesn't bring any financial benefit for the doctor (21%), and can demand extra knowledge and skills (18%). For 12% of the respondents the fact that the effects and benefits of standards are not certain can be a problem for working according to standards.

Table 6. Problems which general practitioners have with working according to standards

	Percentage of respondents agreeing (n=1069)
— old routines are too strong to change	39%
— patients may have other wishes	30%
— medical specialist have other routines	30%
— each patient is different	33%
— may cost extra time or money	29%
— there is no extra financial reward	21%
— lack the right knowledge or skills	18%
— the effects and benefits of standards are uncertain	12%

CONCLUSION

Although there is some positive bias in the data and hough we assessed options and not actual practice performance, within 5 years since the start of the campaign and 3 years after the publication of the first standard, the national standard setting campaign in the Netherlands has been a success among general practitioners. Within one or two years after publication in the College magazine, the great majority of general practitioners are well informed about the existence of the different standards. The College magazine is the most important diffusion channel for informing the doctors about standards. Informal contact with colleagues, CME-activities, and discussing the standards in GP-groups are also very important diffusion channels. Dutch general practitioners think standards are important for the status of the profession and for peer review and educational purposes. Yet many doctors do see some negative influence of standards: they must not become obligatory and there is a chance they can be abused. The overall attitude to national standards is very positive and standards can have a positive effect on daily practice.

To change practice patterns by informing doctors is not enough. The problems doctors can have with 'translating' this information to their own practice setting can vary enormously. In implementing standards in daily practice, it is important to identify individual problems doctors may experience when working according to different standards. These problems can vary from doctor to doctor within GP-groups. Implementation of standards on the level of individual doctors has to take account of these factors and attempt to offer solutions for specific situations. Most of the respondents were very well informed about the different standards and the content of the specific guidelines. Fewer respondents agreed with the guidelines and clearly even fewer respondents said they worked according to these guidelines.

The evaluation of strategies for the implementation of standards and guidelines on regional, local and practice levels will be very important to give information how the acceptance and diffusion of standards and guidelines can have an effect as large as possible.

Making use of different implementation channels, giving doctors support in understanding the meaning of the guidelines, investigating possible problems associated with working according to the different guidelines, and, trying to propose possible solutions for these problems (for instance in discussions in GP-groups), will in the end have the effect that guidelines achieve what they ought to do: be used in daily practice supporting the doctor in his every day work.

REFERENCES

Donabedian A. Criteria and standards for quality assessment and monitoring. *Q R B* 1986; 12: 99-108

Fishbein M, Azjen J. Beliefs, attitudes, intentions and behaviour. Reading: Mass. Addison Wesley Publ. 1975.

Frame P, Kowulich B, Llewellyn A. Improving physician compliance with a health maintenance protocol. *J Fam Pract* 1984; 19: 341-4.

Grol R. National standard setting for quality of care in general practice: attitudes of general practitioners and response to a set of standards. *B J Gen Pract* 1990; 40: 361-4.

Ornstein S, Garr D, et al. Compliance with five health promotion recommendations in a university-based family practice. *J Fam Pract* 1989; 29: 163-8.

Schreiner D, Petrusa E, et.al. Improving compliance with preventive medicine procedures in a house staff training program. *South Med J* 1988; 81: 1553-7.

Selinger H, Goldfarb N, et.al. Physician compliance with mammography guidelines. A retrospective chart review. *Fam Med* 1989; 21: 56-8.

Stange K, Kelly R, et al. Physician agreement with US preventive services task force recommendations. *J Fam Pract* 1992; 34: 409-16.

Yoong A, Lim J, et al. Audit of compliance with ante natal protocols. *BMJ* 1992, 305: 1184-6.

15 Assessing the Quality of an Acute Medicine for the Elderly Service

MARION E. T. McMURDO & DAVID J. GRANT

University of Dundee

INTRODUCTION

Concern about quality is not new, and providers and purchasers of health care are seeking assurance about the quality of health care being provided. For health professionals involved in care which involves a number of practical procedures, quality issues can be tackled in a simple numerical fashion, such as operations performed, or post-operative complications occurring.

For those providing hospital care for the elderly, quality issues are less readily identified. The Dundee Medicine For The Elderly service has 94 assessment beds, and operates a modified age-related service providing rapid admission and assessment for old people with medical problems necessitating in-patient care. The service decided to identify explicit indicators of the quality of its service. A decision was made to select measures which focused on outcome (not on structure or process), and to select tools which were either validated, or could be readily replicated by other units, in order to facilitate inter-unit comparisons.

The elements which constitute a good Medicine For The Elderly Service were identified as follows:

- A Service which returns the majority of its patients to the community
  (i.e. minimises the requirement for longterm hospital or nursing home care.
- A Service which maintains the functional capacity of its elderly patients.
- A Service which plans its discharges in such a way as to minimise unplanned readmissions (less than 28 days after discharge).

METHODS

Our routine structured clerking sheets were altered to include a section on functional status using a modified Barthel Index (Mahoney and Barthel, 1965). In its original form, this functional assessment tool provides a score based on ratings of ability to feed and dress oneself, bathe, go to the toilet, transfer, walk (or propel a wheelchair),

Strategic Issues in Health Care Management. Edited by M. Malek, J. Rasquinha and P. Vacani
© 1993 John Wiley & Sons Ltd

climb stairs, control the bladder and control the bowels. A recent report from Royal College of Physicians and the British Geriatrics Society recommended the Barthel Index in preference over other Activities of Daily Living (ADL) Scales for routine performance of primary ADL (Royal College of Physicians, 1992). This information was recorded by medical staff on admission and discharge in all patients passing through the acute assessment wards of our service. This information, together with data on discharge destination and readmissions were extracted for the case records by a clerkess and recorded on a computerised database designed by ourselves using the DataEase software package.

RESULTS

During the year 1st April 1991 to 31st March 1992, a total of 1087 patients (aged 64-100 years) were discharged from our acute assessment wards. Data were available on 1062/1084 (98%). The mean Barthel score on admission was 77.0 and on discharge was 84.4. The mean modified Barthel scores were 22.2/30 and 24.8/30 respectively. The functional capacity was maintained or improved in 89% of patients for whom data were available.

Excluding deaths, 88.2% of patients were discharged back to the community (either their own home or a residential home) and 11.7% were discharged to long-term care (either nursing home or continuing hospital care).

The total number of readmissions within 28 days was 92, representing a readmission rate of 12%. This data is currently being analysed to distinguish planned from unplanned readmissions, and also to assess the potential preventability of the unplanned readmissions. A total of 71 patients were re-admitted to our unit within 28 days of discharge from other units, mainly the local medical and orthopaedic/trauma units.

DISCUSSION

Quality measurement is an essential step in quality improvement. Measurement difficulties result in a focus on simple measures regardless of whether they are the most critical for quality. The further that quality measures are divorced from outcomes, the greater the risk that they have no real bearing on quality of care.

Current NHS quality assurance initiatives have been criticised for their under-representation of patients' views. The primary purpose of the NHS is, after all, to serve patients. The principal justification for not involving patients in this work is that they do not fully grasp the relevant issues. This project has addressed outcomes which are directly pertinent to elderly patients. Most old (and young) people wish to be restored to living in their own homes, and would reasonably expect to leave hospital in a 'better condition' than they entered it. Although the best tool of its kind, the relative insensitivity of the standard Barthel Index must be acknowledged. Hospital patients are not permitted to bathe unassisted, thus reducing the maximum possible score. In addition, patients who walk independently with a zimmer frame, a stick or without any walking aid sore the same in the appropriate section of the

Barthel, although the aids used reflect different levels of walking ability. In an attempt to address these defects, we modified the Barthel Index for use in hospital inpatients by omitting the sections on bathing, stair climbing, feeding and grooming. In addition, in the remaining sections of dressing, transfers, toileting, continence and mobility, the mobility section has the strongest numerical weighting, reflecting our belief that mobility is the most important of all of these functional characteristics. The Medicine For The Elderly service is picking up a substantial number of 'failed discharges' from other units. This may reflect the pressure to clear beds in the acute units, or an ineptitude among non-geriatricians in dealing with the complex multiple and chronic problems of old age.

This project is, to our knowledge, the first Medicine For The Elderly service to explicitly identify indicators of the quality of its service. Our preliminary work offers the potential for agreement on common standards, and comparisons between different units.

REFERENCES

Mahoney FI and Barthel DW. Functional evaluation: The Barthel Index. Maryland State Medical Journal 1965;14:61-65.

Standardised Assessment Scales For Elderly People. *Royal College of Physicians of London and The British Geriatrics Society*, June 1992.

16 Effectiveness of an Outpatient Geriatric Assessment Unit — Short-Term Results of a Randomized Controlled Study

**VERON J. J. SCHRIJNEMAEKERS &
MEINDERT J. HAVEMAN**

University of Limburg, The Netherlands

INTRODUCTION

In the Netherlands the proportion of elderly in the total population is growing very fast, and this increase will continue in future. In 1991, 12.9% of the Dutch population was 65 years or older (CBS 1992) and prognostic calculations show in the years 2000, 2015 and 2035, percentages will be 14%, 17% and 24% respectively (Ministerie WVC 1990). This makes it necessary to create and evaluate health care services for the elderly.

Several randomized controlled trials (RCT's) of in-patient geriatric assessment units (Allen *et al* 1986; Applegate *et al* 1990; Applegate *et al* 1991; Becker *et al.* 1987; Cole *et al* 1991; Hogan *et al* 1987; Rubenstein *et al* 1984; Rubenstein *et al* 1988; Saltz *et al* 1988) and geriatric programs in the home care setting (Hendriksen *et al* 1984; Van Rossum 1993; Tulloch 1979; Vetter *et al* 1984; Zimmer *et al* 1985) have been done. These experimental studies have demonstrated that geriatric evaluation can lead to improved functional and mental status, more appropriate placement of disabled older persons, decreased use of health care services and reduced mortality.

Less research has been done about effectiveness and efficiency of outpatient geriatric assessment units. In 1987, two controlled experiments of an outpatient multidisciplinary team were executed (Williams *et al* 1987; Yeo *et al* 1987). One study was performed in New York among 117 frail elderly (65+) not residing in an institution (Williams *et al* 1987). The elderly were randomly assigned to receive comprehensive geriatric assessment by a multidisciplinary team (treatment, n=58) or by one of a panel of community internists (controls, n=59). The study showed less hospital days and health care cost for persons with comprehensive geriatric

Strategic Issues in Health Care Management. Edited by M. Malek, J. Rasquinha and P. Vacani
© 1993 John Wiley & Sons Ltd

assessment and there was a trend at 8 months for control subjects to have more functional and mental impairment. The other RCT evaluated a special geriatric clinic staffed by a multidisciplinary team of health professionals with special training in geriatrics, versus a traditional model of general medical clinic care without access to a multidisciplinary team (Yeo *et al* 1987). The results show, among other things, less decline in physical health for the geriatric clinic participants after 18 months.

In light of the results of these studies, and the principle that new services need evaluation, an experiment on the effects of an outpatient geriatric assessment unit (OGA-unit) in the Netherlands was performed. The study was conducted in the Maasland Hospital in Sittard, a town in the South of the Netherlands with 45,000 inhabitants. The main aim of this study is to investigate the preventive effectiveness of the intervention by the OGA-unit on the physical and mental well being of the frail elderly. In this article the first short-term (half year) results are reported.

METHODS

Selection of subjects

The study population was restricted to elderly persons (75+) living at home or in the two residential homes. To avoid contamination by other care, subjects living in a nursing home or who received care from the geriatric outpatient and/or in-patient geriatric unit in the two years before this experiment started were excluded.

To profit from the impact of the OGA-unit, only the physically vulnerable elderly were eligible for this study. In order to make a first selection on vulnerability, a postal questionnaire was send out to all elderly who met the above mentioned criteria and were living at home (n=1207) (figure 1). The response of the elderly to this questionnaire was, after two reminders, 85 percent. Questions were asked about demographic features, activities of daily living (ADL), household activities (IADL), frequency of falls and dizziness, digression of functioning and use of outpatient (in-formal help. Persons with physical problems were defined in this study as a 'high risk' population (29%). Next, these 'high risk' elderly living at home and all the residents of two homes for the elderly were approached for interview by trained interviewers (n=12). Only the elderly who met the criteria for fragility (see appendix 1), and who gave their informed consent to follow-up interviews as well as permission to inform their general practitioner about the results of the interview, were finally included in the study (n=222).

To enhance the prognostic comparability among the contrasted groups, the participants were pre-stratified by living condition, and at home versus In a home for the elderly. The elderly were randomly allocated to the intervention and control group by the researcher. To ensure that the intake at the OGA-unit was gradual, within each stratum a blocked randomization scheme was applied with 10 persons in every block. After randomization, informed consent was asked for persons within the intervention group by their general practitioner (Zelen, 1979). The total selection process (first postal questionnaire to last randomization) took two years (March 1988 – March 1990).

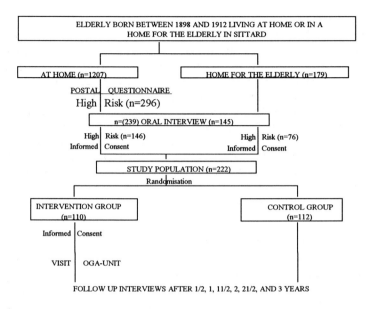

Figure 1. Design Experiment

Intervention

The OGA-unit is meant for elderly who have physical, psychological and/or social complaints. The tasks of the unit are observation, assessment and evaluation to give advice to the general practitioner and the patient concerning treatment and support. At the service, three disciplines are working together namely geriatrics, psychology and social work.

The intervention group (n=110) was offered a comprehensive assessment program in an outpatient geriatric unit. The elderly in the control group (n=112) were not invited for a visit to the OGA-unit. However, they could apply for, or use, all the regular services as before.

Of the 110 frail elderly who were invited to visit the OGA-unit, 56 persons did attend the outpatient clinic. Of the 54 persons who did not attend 8 were not referred by the general practitioner to the unit, 2 died before the intervention took place and 46 elderly refused to go to the geriatric unit. The non response was higher among the elderly who lived in a home for the elderly (60%) than among the elderly at home (46%). From the non response analysis it can be concluded that there were no differences between responders and non-responders in demographic, psychological and social features and in the use of services in the past 6 months. Only physical condition shows statistically significant differences. It appears that the elderly who did not go to the OGA-unit had more (I)ADL limitations and were less mobile. It is possible that limited mobility was a reason not to visit the OGA-unit.

Of the elderly who visited the OGA-unit everybody consulted the geriatrician, 70% were visited at home by the social worker, 17% saw the psychologist and 96%, 76% and 52% respectively had a blood-test, an electrocardiogram and a X-ray. On the basis of the above mentioned assessment an advise, as a written report, was given to the elderly and his GP. For twelve persons (22%), an extended report of all the findings but no additional advise was given. The other 42 elderly received 87 advises. Many advises related to the intake (stop, start or change) of medication (41%), referral to other specialist (14%) or physiotherapist (12%) and with diet (6%).

Some months after the advice the GP was asked whether (s)he followed the advice of the OGA-unit (100% response). It showed that 61% of the advises were (partly) acted upon, and 23% of the recommendations were not followed, in 10% of the cases the GP did not remember what (s)he did and to 10% of the advises the GP could not respond because of the patient's death.

Follow-up and outcome measures

For measuring the effect of the geriatric clinic all elderly in the study population were, as far as possible, approached for 6 follow-up interviews every half year by the same interviewer. This paper discussed the first short-term (½ year) results.

Because mortality will be analysed in this study as an outcome measure in the long run, this article about short-term effects will be restricted to the outcome measures with regard to the physical and psychological well being, such as activities of daily living (ADL-score), household activities (IADL-score), dizziness, falls, mobility, incontinence and vision, as well as depressive (Zung-score) and cognitive complaints (AMT-score).

Statistical analysis

Statistical analyses were performed on the basis of the 'intention to treat' principle. Thus, all patients remain in the group to which they are assigned by randomization. No interim analyses of possible effects for the two groups were published during the intervention period. This was done, to prevent bias in the intervention (OGA-unit) and/or outcome measures (follow-up interviews) by knowing these results.

First, in this article, the comparability at baseline for the two groups and the response for the first half year follow-up will be described. For some outcome measures (ADL, IADL, Zung, AMT) the differences between the follow-up score (t_1) and the baseline score (t_0) were computed. Both groups are compared for differences in their mean scores at the follow-up measurements and also for their mean improvement or deterioration score. For both mean differences, 90 percent confidence limits were calculated. For the other dichotomous outcome measures the percentages at the start and after a half year are given for both groups. For the differences in percentages between the intervention and control group, a 90 percent confidence interval was computed. The analyses were carried out with SPSS-PC (Norusis 1990) and BMDP (Dixon *et al* 1990).

RESULTS

Comparability at baseline

To check whether the randomization has resulted in two comparable groups, baseline data have been compared for the intervention and control group (appendix 2).Besides the living condition, which the elderly had been stratified on, the majority of the prognostic characteristics showed no considerable differences.

The intervention group appeared to include more men (66% vs 74%) and some more married elderly (65% vs 77%) than in the control group. The other demographic variables were almost identically distributed for both groups. With respect to the physical characteristics the differences were nearly nil. With regard to the psychological data, it arose that the presence of depressive complaints (≥ 60) was statistically significant higher in the intervention group ($\chi^2=5.4$; p=0.02). However, the mean Zung-score (53.3 vs 50.9) showed no statistical significant difference (t=-1.33; p=0.2). Also, when other cutpoints (50, 55 and 65) were chosen for identifying depressive complaints, none of them showed statistically significant differences ($\chi^2 = 0.47$, p=0.5; $\chi^2 1.8$, p=0.2; $\chi^2=0.61$, p=0.4) anymore between both groups. Except for consultation with the GP, the use of health care services were at the baseline almost comparable for both groups. In general it can be stated that the resemblance of both groups at the start appeared to be satisfactory.

Mortality and non-participation

Mortality is considered as an outcome measure in the long run of this experiment. However, mortality is also of potential influence for the other outcome measures. For this reason, it is important to describe the nonresponse due to mortality or other reasons precisely. Other reasons of nonresponse are non-participation of elderly who could not or would not be interviewed after six months (t_1). In table 1 the figures of non-participation are given. The response rate at t_1 was 82%, 7% of the elderly died and 11% did not participate because of other reasons. In the first half year of the trial death as well as nonresponse, appeared more often in the intervention group. Although, these findings are not statistically significant a potential bias could be introduced by selection.

Table.1 Percentages (non-)response after six months in the intervention and control group

	Intervention (n=110)		Control (n=112)		Total (n=222)	
	%	n	%	n	%	n
response	77	(85)	87	(97)	82	(182)
died	9	(10)	5	(5)*	7	(15)
nonresponse	14	(15)	9	(10)**	11	(25)

*   90% Confidence Interval: (-2% / 10%)
**   90% Confidence Interval: (-2% / 12%)

For this reason respondents and non-respondents are compared in some baseline characteristics. This comparison is done separately for the intervention and control group. The number of persons in each group at the baseline is showed in table 2.

Table 2. Baseline characteristics (means) for (non-) respondents
intervention (I) and control (C) group

	Response (n=182)		Dropout * (n=40)		Died (n=15)		Non-response (n=25)	
	I	C	I	C	I	C	I	C
Age	81.9	82.3	82.8	81.3	84.5	79.4[1]	81.6	82.3
ADL-score	1.2	1.2	1.5	3.2[2]	2.0	4.0	1.2	2.9
IADL-score	4.7	4.5	5.3	6.5	6.1	7.4	4.9	6.1
Zung-score	53.3	51.0	53.4	50.7	53.8	45.0	53.2	53.7
AMT-score	8.3	8.6	7.6	6.7	7.8	8.0	7.5	6.2

  * dropout=died+nonresponse   1 t=-2.4; p=0.03   2 t=-2.1; p=0.05

It appears from the figures in table 2 that the differences between the intervention and control group for the response group are small (columns 1 & 2). But looking more specifically, dropouts (columns 3 & 4) had more physical limitations ((I)ADL) and mental complaints (AMT) than the respondents (column 1 & 2). Considering the dropouts only (columns 3 & 4) persons of the control group had statistically significant higher ADL-scores than the elderly in the intervention group.

It seems that there are some differences in nonresponse between the intervention and control group at the first follow-up interview. Because there is no suitable method to control for this, and because of the small baseline differences for the persons who completed the first follow-up, we decided to restrict the analysis to only those elderly who completed the t_0 and t_1 interview (n=182).

Short-term outcome measures

Table 3 shows the mean scores on (I)ADL, Zung and AMT at the start and after six months for the intervention and control group. The mean changes over time for both groups are presented in the same table. Changes in mean score (last column) are calculated at the individual level.

A negative difference for the ADL, IADL and Zung means that the intervention group had a lower, and thus a more favourable score compared to the control group. The opposite applies to the AMT score. At first sight the mean scores and the mean changes in score over time do not seem to relate logically. This discrepancy is caused by the fact that the change in mean score could only be calculated for those subjects who had no missing value in both measurements (individual level) and the mean score is computed on group level. Almost no short-term differences are found concerning the functional status (ADL and IADL score). Both groups have a very small decrease in their physical functioning. However, the small differences found were in favour of the intervention group.

Table 3. Mean scores and mean changes in scores in the intervention (n=85) and control group (n=97) (90% CI)

	mean scores				mean changes			
	I*	C*	difference	90% CI	I*	C*	difference	90% CI
ADL-score								
start	1.2	1.2	0.0	(-0.4/0.4)				
½ year	1.3	1.4	-0.1	(-0.6/0.4)	+0.1	+0.2	-0.1	(-0.4/+0.2)
IADL-score								
start	4.7	4.5	+0.2	(-0.3/0.7)				
½ year	4.9	4.8	+0.1	(-0.4/0.7)	+0.2	+0.3	-0.1	(-0.6/+0.2)
Zung-score								
start	53.3	51.0	+2.3	(-1.0/5.6)				
½ year	49.7	52.4	-2.7	(-6.0/0.6)	-3.4	+1.6	-5.0	(-7.5/-2.4)
AMT-score								
start	8.3	8.6	-0.3	(-0.8/0.2)				
½ year	8.6	8.5	+0.1	(-0.4/0.6)	+0.3	0.1	+0.4	(0.0/+0.7)

* I=intervention   C=control

Concerning the depressive complaints (Zung score) there is a statistically significant result in favour of the elderly in the intervention group. Whereas a decrease of the mean Zung score (-3.4) was found for the elderly in the intervention group in the first half year, an increase (+1.6) was found for persons of the control group. The difference between the two groups (-5.0) has a confidence interval that does not include the zero, which means that the mean difference is statistically significant. Additionally it appeared that many of the single Zung-items (n=14) showed a change in favour of the intervention group. This is enough evidence that there are no specific components of the Zung-scale which take account for the differences, but that depressive complaints in general differ between the two groups.

The AMT score (cognitive problems) shows also a difference in favour of the elderly who visited the OGA-unit but does not reach statistical significance. Additionally, a one-way analysis of covariance (ANCOVA), was performed to estimate the differences in the mean score by adjusting for the difference between the two groups at the start with regard to the outcome measure in question and for some demographic variables (gender, marital status and age). These results vary only marginally from the figures in table 3.

In table 4, a negative difference implies a favourable score (less limitations) for the intervention group. For both groups there is a decrease of dizziness and falls in the first half year of the experiment. In this same period there is also a reduction of mobility, and it is possible that elderly who walk less have a smaller risk to fall or become dizzy. An alternative explanation is the regression to the mean phenomenon. But if this is the case, than a decrease in the same order should be found for other indicators of fragility, as well, and with the same impact for both groups. The decline in dizziness and incontinence is, however, in favour of the intervention group. In the first half years almost no changes with regard to visual impairment appeared in both groups.

Table 4. Percentages physical limitations and their changes in the first half year in the intervention (n=85) and control group (n=97)

	I%	C%	difference	90% CI	% of change I	C	difference
Dizziness: often							
start	52	52	0	(-0.12,0.12)			
½ year	31	42	-11	(-0.23,0.01)	-21	-10	-11
Falls: > 1×							
start	39	45	-6	(-0.18,0.06)			
½ year	20	27	-7	(-0.17,0.03)	-19	-18	-1
Walking distance: 0/indoors							
start	44	41	3	(-0.09,0.15)			
½ year	49	45	4	(-0.08,0.16)	5	4	1
Incontinence							
start	39	44	-5	(-0.17,0.07)			
½ year	30	40	-10	(-0.22,0.02)	-9	-4	-5
Read text TV: sometimes/no							
start	46	43	3	(0.09,0.15)			
½ year	41	41	0	(-0.12,0.12)	-5	-2	-3
Read newspaper: sometimes/no							
start	39	38	1	(-0.11,0.13)			
½ year	39	40	-1	(-0.13,0.11)	0	2	2

DISCUSSION

In general, the short term impact of the outpatient geriatric assessment unit on the health status of frail elderly was limited. Elderly who were assessed by the OGA-unit had almost the same deterioration in their physical abilities after six months than the elderly who received the regular services. There were some exceptions and the small differences which were found, were in favour of the intervention group. Dizziness and incontinence were less prevalent after six months in persons of the OGA-unit.

The results of this study are in line with the findings of the two studies which are most comparable with regard to type of intervention and research design with our study. One of the studies (Williams *et al* 1987) showed more functional impairments after 8 months for control subjects, but this difference was not statistically significant. Significantly less decline in functional health was found for the outpatient geriatric clinic participants in another study after 18 months (Yeo *et al* 1987). Although we cannot confirm this conclusion at this stage, because our long-term figures are not yet analysed, it enlarges our interest in possible long-term effects on physical well-being.

With regard to depressive complaints we found a statistically significant result in favour of the elderly who were asked to visit the OGA-unit. The elderly showed an improvement in their depressive complaints whereas the elderly in the control group had more problems. Yeo's results (1987) concerning depressive complaints were also in favour of the intervention group but did not reach statistical significance. Williams

(1987) states that there was a trend at 8 months for control subjects to have more mental impairment. Possible explanations for the differences in depressive complaints are the following. Respectively 100%, 70% and 17% of the elderly who consulted the OGA-unit, saw a geriatrician, social worker at home and a psychologist at the unit. These disciplines are pre-eminently suitable to assess and advice about treatment of psychological problems. It appeared that the advises of the OGA-unit to the patients and their GP's contained six times an advice about starting an anti-depressant drug.

ACKNOWLEDGEMENT

This project is funded by the Province of Limburg and the Directorate Policy for the Elderly of the Ministry of Social Welfare, Public Health and Cultural Affairs.

APPENDICES

Appendix 1. Selection criteria from interviews

1. Elderly person cannot independently fulfil 5 from the 11 household activities (IADL) <u>and</u> carrying out these activities has become more difficult the last six months. (This criterium does not apply for the elderly of the residential homes)

OR

2. Elderly person cannot independently fulfil 3 from the 12 activities of daily living (ADL) and carrying out the activities has become more difficult the last six months.

OR

3. Elderly person does not reach the toilet in time more often than earlier and finds this inconvenient.

OR

4. Elderly person had a deterioration in mobility and has fallen the last six months more than once or has often troubles with dizziness.

OR

5. The interviewer judges that the interview was very difficult because of serious agitation or confusion from the elderly person.

When the elderly person meets one of the 5 criteria mentioned and furthermore answers the informed consent questions positive, randomization takes place.

Appendix 2. Distribution of baseline characteristics among the intervention and control group

Characteristic		intervention (n=110)		Control (n=112)	
Demographic					
Living Condition	at home	65	(72)	66%	(74)
	residential home	35	(38)	34%	(38)
Gender	female	65	(72)	74%	(83)
	male	35	(38)	26%	(29)
Marital Status	married	35	(38)	23%	(36)
	unmarried	65	(72)	77%	(86)
Age	77-84	69	(76)	71%	(80)
	≥ 85	31	(34)	29%	(32)
Physical					
ADL-score*	0	49	(53)	52%	(57)
	1-9	51	(55)	48%	(52)
IADL-score*	0-3	26	(25)	34%	(35)
	4-8	74	(73)	66%	(67)
dizziness	0/some times	51	(56)	51%	(57)
falls	0-1x	62	(68)	60%	(66)
	> 1x	38	(41)	40%	(44)
walking distance	> 5	55	(60)	55%	(62)
	0/indoors	45	(49)	45%	(50)
incontinence	yes	42	(43)	39%	(42)
	no	58	(59)	61%	(66)
read text t.v.	yes	53	(57)	57%	(63)
	sometimes/no	47	(51)	43%	(47)
read newspaper	yes	46	(68)	62%	(71)
	sometimes/no	36	(41)	38%	(40)
Psychological					
Zung-score*	<60	65	(71)	79%	(89)[1]
	≥ 60	35	(39)	21%	(23)
AMT-score*	0-8	44	(48)	35%	(39)
	9-10	56	(62)	65%	(72)
Use of health care services**					
general practitioner		96	(106)	84%	(94)[2]
specialist		64	(70)	63%	(70)
admission hospital		15	(16)	14%	(16)
physiotherapist		24	(26)	21%	(23)
social worker		12	(13)	6%	(7)
district nurse***		22	(16)	19%	(14)
home help***		50	(36)	37%	(27)

          1. $\chi^2=5.4$; p=0.02   2. $\chi^2=9.6$; p=0.002

   *   See appendix 2 for the operationalization of the characteristics
  **   Last half year
 ***   Concerning the independently living elderly only

Appendix 3. Some research variables and their operationalization

Variable	Operationalization	Scores (range and Cronbach's α)
ADL-score	Sum of disabilities in 9 activities of daily living: eating/drinking; in/out chair; toileting; washing hands/face; mobility indoors; in/out bed; dressing; putting on shoes/socks; bathing	0-9, α =.86
IADL-score	Sum of disabilities in 8 household activities: making lunch; wash up; cooking; managing money; making beds; shopping; laundering; mopping/washing windows	0-8, α =.76
Zung-score*	Index score from the "Depressive Status Inventory" (DSI) (Zung, 1972): (The item "I feel that others would be better off if I were dead" was erased)	25-100, α =.82
AMT-score**	"Abbreviated Mental Test" (AMT) (Qureshi, 1972)	0-10, α =.80

Note: the underlined score indicates the most favourable score for each scale.
*index-scores of 60 or higher are indicative of depressive complaints
**scores of 8 or higher are indicative of memory disturbance

REFERENCES

Allen, C.M., Becker, P.M., McVey, L.J., Saltz, C., Feussner, J.R. and Cohen H.J. (1986), 'A randomized, controlled clinical trial of a geriatric consultation team', *JAMA*, 19, 2617-2621.

Applegate, W.B., Miller, S.T., Graney, M.J., Elam, J.T., Burns, R. and Akins, D.E. (1990), 'A randomized, controlled trial of a geriatric assessment unit in a community rehabilitation hospital', *The New England Journal of Medicine*, 22, 1572-1578.

Applegate, W.B., Graney, M.J., Miller, S.T. and Elam, J.T. (1991), 'Impact of a geriatric assessment unit on subsequent health care charges', *American Journal of Public Health*, 10, 1302-1306.

Becker, P.M., McVey, L.J., Saltz, C.C., Feussner, J.R. and Cohen, H.J. (1987), 'Hospital-acquired complications in a randomized controlled clinical trial of a geriatric consultation team', *JAMA*, 17, 2313-2317.

Centraal Bureau voor de Statistiek (1992), *Statistisch Jaarboek 1992*, Voorburg/Heerlen.

Cole, M.G., Fenton, F.R., Engelsmann, F. and Mansouri, I. (1991), 'Effectiveness of geriatric psychiatry consultation in an acute care hospital: a randomized clinical trial', *JAGS*, 39, 1183-1188.

Dixon, W.J., Broun, M.B., Engelmann, L. and Jennrich, R.I. (1990), *BMDP statistical software manual*, University of California Press, Berkeley.

Hendriksen, C., Lund, E. and Strømård, E. (1984), 'Consequences of assessment and intervention among elderly people: a three year randomized controlled trial', *British Medical Journal* 289, 1522-1524.

Hogan, D.B., Fox, R.A., Badley, B.W.D. and Mann, O.E. (1987), 'Effect of a geriatric consultation service on management of patients in an acute care hospital', *CMAJ*, 136, 713-717.

Ministerie van WVC (1990), *Verkenning van de veroudering in Nederland*, Rijswijk.

Norusis, M.J. (1990), *SPSS Statistical data analysis*, SPSS Inc., Chicago.

Qureshi, K.N. and Hodkinson, H.M. (1972), 'Evaluation of a ten-question mental test in the institutionalized elderly', *Age and Ageing*, 3, 152-157.

Rossum van, E. (1993), *Effects of preventive home visits to the elderly*, PhD thesis, Maastricht (in press).

Rubenstein, L.Z., Josephson, K.R., Wieland, G.D., English, P.A., Sayre, J.A. and Kane, R.L. (1984), 'Effectiveness of a geriatric evaluation unit; a randomized clinical trial', *New England Journal of Medicine* 26, 1664-1670.

Rubenstein, L.Z., Wieland, G.D., Josephson, K.R., Rosbrook, B., Sayre, J. and Kane, R.L. (1988), 'Improved survival for frail elderly inpatients on a geriatric evaluation unit (GEU): Who benefits?', *Journal of Clinical Epidemiology*, 5, 441-449.

Saltz, C.C., McVey, L.J., Becker, P.M., Feussner, J.R. and Cohen, H.J. (1988), 'Impact of a geriatric consultation team on discharge placement and repeat hospitalization', *The Gerontologist* 3, 344-350.

Tulloch, A.J. (1979), 'A randomized controlled trial of geriatric screening and surveillance in general practice', *Journal of the Royal College of General Practitioners* 29, 733-742.

Vetter, N.J., Jones, D.A. and Victor, C.R. (1984), 'Effect of health visitors working with elderly patients in general practice: a randomized controlled trial', *British Medical Journal* 288, 369-372.

Williams, M.E., Williams, T.F., Zimmer, J.G., Hall, W.J. and Podgorski, C.A. (1987), 'How does the team approach to outpatient geriatric evaluation compare with traditional care: a report of a randomized controlled trial', *JAGS* 12, 1071-1078.

Yeo, G., Ingram, L., Skurnick, J. and Crapo, L. (1987), 'Effects of a geriatric clinic on functional health and well-being of elders', *Journal of Gerontology* 3, 252-258.

Zelen, M. (1979), 'A new design for randomized clinical trials', *New England Journal of Medicine* 22, 1242-1245.

Zimmer, J.G., Groth-Juncker, A. and McCusker, J. (1985), 'A randomized controlled study of a home health care team', *AJPH* 2, 134-141.

Zung, W.W.K. (1972), 'The depression status inventory: an adjunct to the self-rating depression scale', *Journal of Clinical Epidemiology* 28, 539-543.

17 Linking Clinical Reality with Strategic Management

VALERIE ILES, DEREK CRAMP & EWART CARSON

City University, London

INTRODUCTION

A scan of the Thursday and Sunday quality newspapers in any week in the United Kingdom will reveal advertisements for Managing Directors of manufacturing companies; all of them specifying manufacturing or production experience as a requirement. In a similar vein, newly graduated MBAs lament the fact that companies will not take them seriously unless they have sector specific experience. Furthermore, it is unusual to find chief executives of any large commercial company who have not spent a significant period in its leading functions - often sales and marketing in addition to the core business. In the U.S.A. this philosophy extends to the health care sector where many hospitals are now run by dual qualified chief-executives: doctors with an MBA.

Prior to the Griffiths Report (Griffiths, 1983) the consensus management team at the pinnacle of Health Authority organisational structures consisted of members of the two dominant clinical professions, medicine and nursing, and the guardians of the Authority's means of obtaining its finances - the chief Administrator and Treasurer. These could be considered the leading functions, and between them they brought to strategic management decisions an essential knowledge of operational detail. If management by consensus sometimes became management by veto it was not because the system *could* not work, but because small politics intervened so that it *would* not work. The implementation of the Griffiths Report (Griffiths, 1983) introduced 'General Management' - the instatement of the "one person in charge". Florence Nightingale's lamp could now return to its rightful use.[1]

Finding individuals with experience of those three leading functions was of course impossible. Doctors and nurses were encouraged to apply but about 90% of Unit and District General Manager posts went to ex-administrators or managers from outside

---

[1] Griffiths: *if Florence Nightingale were alive with her lamp today she would assuredly be using it to try and find out who's in charge*

Strategic Issues in Health Care Management. Edited by M. Malek, J. Rasquinha and P. Vacani
© 1993 John Wiley & Sons Ltd

health care. In the fullness of time the term 'administrator' disappeared to be replaced by the term 'manager'. The resulting anomaly is that most of the people in the NHS who manage the link between resources displayed and services delivered do not consider themselves managers but clinicians; and most of the people who are called managers do not *manage* anything but support others in *their* management task.

The internal market has increased the importance (to health care *organisations*) of strategic management decisions being well-informed. Thus chief executives must understand enough about the operational detail of their organisation (the clinical issues) to commission, interpret or evaluate that information. It is the intention of this paper to show that one of the major inhibitors of effective strategic decision making in health care is lack of understanding at senior management level of clinical issues. This results in a lack of credibility of managers in the eyes of their clinical colleagues, which further compounds the problem. What is needed is a shared perception of, and commitment to, corporate objectives which can only be achieved when managers and clinicians understand each other's priorities.

CLINICAL REALITY — OPERATIONAL MANAGEMENT IN HEALTH CARE

Models of service organisation

Sasser (1978) describes two extremes on a spectrum of service organisation types. He calls them the Consumer Service Organisation (CSO) and the Professional Service Organisation (PSO). McDonalds is an example of a CSO and McKinsey's management consultancy a PSO. The CSO produces a standard product or range of products, employs cheap, unqualified staff, with good social skills but no interest in decision making. There is a high turnover of staff. Decisions are taken centrally and there is very limited local autonomy.

In the PSO, staff members are highly qualified (through education and experience) and each makes a significant contribution to the activities of the organisation as a whole. Each project undertaken is individually tailored to the needs of the client and these must first be diagnosed. The PSO staff are expensive, they are encouraged to stay and turnover is low. Few decisions are taken centrally. There is much autonomy for staff members. Managers are more generalist than the specialists they manage and provide support in terms of approach rather than detail. They monitor performance in terms of successful completion of projects and repeat business, and are not concerned with what time of day the work is undertaken as long as it is done.

Clearly most health care organisations (providers certainly) contain sub-organisations which tend toward the CSO end of the spectrum (cleaning, catering) and others which are PSOs (the medical profession and some of the Professions Allied to Medicine (PAMs), with others, e.g. nursing, somewhere in the middle). It must be recognised that the role of senior managers in relation to these different sub-sets must be different. This may seem obvious, but how often does one hear of the manager in charge of car-parking, porters, laundry, estates, catering and domestics being "given" the PAMs to manage!?

Donabedian (1977) discussed the concepts of structure, process and outcome in relation to clinical care. He defined these as:

- Structure   — the structures and systems in place (including a system of medical audit, for example); also premises, heating etc
- Process   — the interaction between clinician and client
- Outcome   — the clinical state of client as a result of intervention

However, it is helpful to refine this analysis and consider structure, process and outcome for the manager, clinician, and client, respectively.

Manager in the health care provider organisation

Structure
- money,
- professional and other kinds of expertise and skills, in the form of staff employed or available for employment by the organisation,
- requirement to treat a certain number and case mix of clients,
- premises, owned or available for purchase,
- equipment, owned or available for purchase.

Process
- setting up all the systems, employing the right people, taking decisions to enter or withdraw from particular markets or activities.

Outcome
- CSO elements   — work well in terms of product quality assurance and consumer satisfaction.
- PSO elements   — staff have skills, resources and motivation to diagnose and meet the client's needs.

Clinicians

Structure — the structures and systems in place
Process — the diagnosis of the client's needs, appraisal of treatment options available, recommendations for treatment.
Outcome — client is informed about, and supported in, decisions about treatment, and also in compliance with treatment.

Clients

Structure — consultation, information about clinical condition and treatment options.
Process — treatment.

Outcome — change of clinical status as a result of treatment.

Whether we consider the Sasser definition of a PSO, or consider the structure/process/outcome concerns of managers, clinicians, and clients, we can clearly see that there are elements of the clinical role (those elements that take place between clinician and client) in which the manager cannot intervene on a case-by-case basis. However, even here there will be norms in terms of approach and it is within the manager's remit to ensure that these norms are adhered to.

Medical Audit has been claimed by the medical profession and managers often agree, that there is no role for them in this wholly professional activity. This is an example of managers understepping the mark. It is legitimate for them to require that standards are set, for them to know what the standards are, for them to agree the methods used to monitor performance against those standards, and to know the results of that monitoring. They also have a right to know what changes in practice are planned as a result of the monitoring.

If this is an example of managers understepping the mark there are plenty of instances of their overstepping it. For instance, when a mental health trust chief executive over-rules a consultant psychiatrist over an admission decision; or when a hospital trust requires its consultants to reduce the number of follow-up visits in out-patients. If managers are to manage at an operational level in health care they must be sufficiently knowledgeable about the clinical role to know what decisions are properly clinical and which are managerial.

STRATEGIC MANAGEMENT

The essence of strategic management is ensuring the best fit between the internal resources of an organisation and its external environment. This involves making decisions about what markets to be in, and how to compete in those markets. Any appraisal of the internal resources and their comparative strengths and weaknesses requires an inside-out understanding of the organisation, its staff, its systems, its technology, and so on.

To many general managers any systems that relate to clinical procedures, clinical equipment, clinical practices and clinical developments are a closed book; but it is in this operational detail that competitive advantage lies. Without an understanding of this detail how can a senior manager assess whether trends and events in the external environment afford opportunities to be seized, or whether defensive action may be required? In the acute sector, care is a high technology affair and such technology does not come cheaply. How can managers make a robust appraisal of different technological options, if they are dependent on clinicians for key data projections and have no means of testing those assumptions?

More and more, managers are taking 'make or buy' decisions. Clearly these decisions require a sound grasp of business economics, but they also pre-suppose a good understanding of the areas under consideration. Without this operational insight and detailed knowledge of the organisation, the tools and techniques of strategic management can be applied only superficially. This has two outcomes: one is that the decisions taken on the basis of these analyses are sub-optimal, and the other is that when the analyses are made available to clinical staff they perceive the analytical tools to be at fault. This further diminishes, for them, the credibility of the body of knowledge held by managers and hence managers themselves.

GENERAL MANAGERS VERSUS REAL MANAGERS

Let us accept that there is a legitimate and valuable administrative function that enables health care organisations to operate efficiently and effectively. It is clear that people fulfilling this function now call themselves general managers. Many administrators are also real managers, as many nurses, therapists, and doctors are also real managers in the sense that they achieve their own objectives through other people. It must, however, be clearly understood that becoming a real manager (whatever the professional background) requires different skills, knowledge and behaviour. For real managers to really manage services outside their own professional domain they must develop an understanding of the operational issues right across their new area of responsibility.

Why is this distinction important? There are several reasons. Firstly, if we confuse management with administration we devalue the administrative role and fail to provide appropriate training and career paths. Health care organisations are currently using the administration skills of individuals trained and developed in a previous era. We are in danger of not replacing those skills.

Secondly, if management is equated with administration we shall never attract doctors in particular to senior real management posts. As always, the politically correct term acquires the value of the non-politically correct term it replaces (apparently playground humour now includes the epithet 'L.D.' — short for learning difficulty, used in the same way as the old 'mentally deficient' or 'mentally handicapped' phases). This is important because, as we have demonstrated above, we need clinical professionals in top management positions — not to manage other doctors in place of a general manager who is opting out of that function (which is what clinical directorates are concerned with) — but because they know more about the intricacies of a complex system than almost anyone else.

THE DEVELOPMENT OF REAL MANAGERS

Real managers need an understanding of clinical issues, the financial and administrative framework, and management concepts, tools and behaviours. Since no recognised career pattern exists to produce such individuals, appropriate education and development programmes must be devised.

Provision of the factual input regarding the financial and administrative framework is relatively straightforward. Management education is far from straightforward as it involves a shift in attitude as much as an acquisition of knowledge; however many centres have developed expertise in this area. It is nevertheless worth stressing that running short management courses for clinicians, with a superficial introduction to a number of tools, without adequate explanation of the principles behind them, and without demonstration of the quality and clarity of thought required in their use, does more harm than good.

The more challenging aspect is the engendering of clinical insight, and an interest in clinical issues and developments, in those with no clinical background. It is not, after all, possible to teach all of medicine, nursing, physiotherapy, radiography, dietetics etc, and nor would one want to.

Management educators have distilled the principles of accounting and economics, for example, to teach managers how to interact effectively with accountants and economists. We need to do the same. This must involve:

- key elements of the clinical task, clinical starting points (the human body and populations), clinical process, clinical decision making.
- key requirements, constraints and potential outcomes of the clinical professions (pre-and post-registration education, registration).
- clinical language.

We also need to convey the niceties of the elite club to which doctors belong, with its different grades of membership and the mechanisms by which members gain and lose status within it. This is not easy and must involve a mixture of factual input, learning different perspectives on issues at the clinical/managerial interface, role play, shadowing opportunities and debate with active practitioners.

In the Health Management Group at City University we have developed a Masters degree in Health Management in which we attempt to do this (Iles, 1992).

CLAIMING THE CONCEPT OF MANAGEMENT

In addition to the development of individuals with the skills and insight required of real managers, a nationwide debate is needed to identify the managerial elements of the role of senior clinicians.

Management as a concept must also be reclaimed. This will mean laying to rest some of the myths that surround management. Senior professionals need to be reassured that managing people does not mean telling them what to do and then policing them. It will, however, involve agreeing objectives and being a resource to others in the achievement of those objectives. It also requires meaningful sanctions when agreed objectives are not achieved. This needs full and frank discussions and a robust on going relationship. In this way we must enthuse high calibre health professionals into top real management roles and once again ensure that strategic management decisions are rooted in clinical reality.

REFERENCES

Donabedian, A. (1977), Explorations in Quality Assessment and Monitoring. Vol I Definitions of Quality and Approaches to its Assessment, Health Administration Press, Ann Arbor, Michigan.

Griffiths, R. (1983), NHS Management Inquiry (The Griffiths Report), Department of Health and Social Security, London.

Iles, V.M. (1992), The importance of talking shop, Health Service Journal, March 1992.

Sasser, W.E. (1978) Management of Service Operations, Allys and Bacon, Boston, Mass.

Section IV

Hospital and Community Care

18 More Market, Less Competition and More Strategy in the Hospital Market

RICHARD JANSSEN & MARTIN DEN HARTOG

University of Limburg, The Netherlands

INTRODUCTION

Dutch health care reforms are intended to introduce more market-oriented structures. Competition between health care insurers is expected to improve efficiency. In addition, health care insurers should buy health care services more efficiently. As Porter (1988) stated, competition in an industry depends on five basic forces: rivalry among existing competitors, the bargaining power of buyers and suppliers, the threat of new entrants, and the presence of substitute products.

In this paper we will examine to what extent three of these forces; i.e. rivalry among suppliers, the bargaining power of buyers and the threat of new entrants, contribute to competition in the hospital services market. The paper begins with a short description of the Dutch health care system and the proposed health care reforms. Porter's model, which serves as an analytical tool to systematize developments in the market for hospital services is then introduced. The empirical section of the paper presents figures showing the process of concentration in the hospital market. Various concentration indices are used in this study to measure this process. The same approach is then used to describe the structure of the health insurance market followed by a comparison of the bargaining powers of insurers and hospitals. The threat of new entrants is then empirically investigated. The subject of strategic management is discussed, and a short survey of the literature of some possible future developments with the help of the dynamic theory of the market (De Jong 1989) is examined. Several strategies are discussed, such as backward integration by insurers, forward integration by suppliers, and diversification and specialisation by hospitals.

Strategic Issues in Health Care Management. Edited by M. Malek, J. Rasquinha and P. Vacani
© 1993 John Wiley & Sons Ltd

THE NETHERLANDS MARKET FOR HOSPITAL SERVICES

Some system characteristics of the health care system

It is common practice to categorise health care systems according to three basic models: the national health service model, the social (or statutory) insurance model and the private insurance model. The Dutch system could be described as a combination of social insurance and private insurance (Janssen and van der Made 1991). The insurance system is composed of three elements: the Exceptional Medical Expenses Act, the Sickness Funds Insurance Act, and private insurance schemes.

The Exceptional Medical Expenses Act (AWBZ) provides social insurance for all Dutch citizens. This compulsory insurance scheme covers exceptional medical expenses such as admissions to nursing homes or institutions for the handicapped, prolonged stays in hospitals and so on. It is financed mainly by income-related contributions. In the past the AWBZ was operated by public health insurance companies, known as Sickness Funds, but now, as part of the reforms, the private insurers have been included in the operation of the AWBZ. The Sickness Funds are voluntary non-profit organisations.

The Sickness Funds Insurance Act (Ziekenfondswet) covers short term care and is compulsory for wage-earners and social security beneficiaries with an income below a certain level. About 62% of the population is insured under the Sickness Funds Insurance Act, which is operated by the Sickness Funds. The premium is proportional to gross income up to a ceiling. There are about 40 regional Sickness Funds, and an employee must choose a fund in his or her geographic region.

Students, the self-employed, and the 32% of the population who earn more than 55,000 guilders have to arrange private insurance for the risks that are not covered by the AWBZ. The premiums they pay are in general risk-related. They may opt out of insurance for part of their health care and accept higher deductibles in return for premium reductions. These insurance schemes are offered by private insurers, some of whom are non-profit organisations. The remaining 6% of the population are civil servants, who work for the national, regional or local governments and are covered under a separate plan. In this plan premiums are income-related and co-payments are part of employment conditions.

The premiums for the exceptional medical expenses scheme and the mandatory Sickness Fund premiums cover about 65% of the total expenditure of health care. The government budget contributes about 10% and the remaining 25% comes from private contributions and direct payments from patients. So the financing system in the Netherlands is a mix of public and private insurance, and relies partly on employer contributions.

Table 1 shows the spread of total health care financing over the various funds. The share of the Sickness Funds has decreased, in contrast to expenditures under the Special Sickness Expenses Act, which have increased, especially since 1989. This is caused by the addition of extra mural psychiatric treatment to the AWBZ scheme. The share borne by government funds went up to about 15% in the mid

1980s and decreased to around 10% in the early 1990s. Total public expenditures, including the costs of statutory insurance schemes, stabilized at between 70% and 75% of the total in the 1980s.

Table 1. Percentage of expenditure financed by different funds

	1975	1985	1986	1987	1988	1989	1990	1991	1992[a]	1993[a]
Sickness Insurance Act	42.5	36.5	34.9	35.1	35.2	32.4	32.5	33.1	26.4	26.4
Special Sickness Expenses Act	24.0	23.3	23.1	23.8	23.7	30.5	31.2	31.1	40.8	41.5
Government	7.2	15.0	15.2	13.8	13.5	10.2	10.5	10.3	10.3	10.3
Private Resources	26.3	25.2	26.8	27.3	27.5	26.9	25.7	25.5	22.5	21.8
Costs per Capita	1338	2836	2926	3016	3053	3052	3093	3498	3619	3704
Costs % of GNP	10.3%	9.8%	10.0%	10.1%	9.9%	9.6%	9.6%	9.8%	9.8%	9.8%

[a] Estimate

Source: *Financial Survey of Health Care*, various volumes

The provision of health care facilities in the Netherlands is predominantly non-public. Hospitals and other intramural[1] institutions are voluntary associations and can therefore be characterised as private non-profit organizations.

Under the terms of the Hospital Facilities Act (*Wet Ziekenhuisvoorzieningen*) the government plans the capacity and distribution of intramural health care facilities such as hospitals and nursing homes. The issue of the payment of hospitals will be discussed later.

Specialist care is generally provided in hospitals. Both publicly and privately insured patients receive treatment in the same hospitals, although private patients claim extra facilities, and pay an additional premium.

Remuneration of suppliers

The inpatient and outpatient services of specialists are charged separately from the hospital budget on a fee-for-service basis. Physicians, whether hospital-based or in private practice, and other medical professionals work as free commercial entrepreneurs. The total costs of specialist care amount to about 5.5% of total health care costs in the Netherlands.

General practitioners receive a capitation fee for each publicly insured patient on their list (Groenewegen et al 1991). They receive a full tariff for the first 1,600 patients and a lower tariff for any additional patients. GPs are paid on a fee-for-service basis by privately insured patients. Practically all GPs have both publicly and privately insured patients. GP services receive about 5% of total health care expenditure. Over 90% of the GPs operate from private offices, working as independent contractors under the health insurance scheme. Some 7% work in

---

[1] Health care services are divided into 'intramural' and 'extramural' services. Intramural services are all services delivered within the walls of a hospital or residential institution, thus including non-admission departments such as Accident and Emergency and Outpatients. All other services are 'extramural'.

health centres, but only one-third of these GPs are employed by the health centre rather than being self-employed. Publicly insured clients need a referral from a GP for a consultation with a medical specialist, so that GPs can be considered as the gate-keepers of the health care system.

In addition, some services such as community health services, and sometimes also hospitals, are publicly (municipally) owned. They account for about 3% of the total health care expenditure.

Pharmaceuticals are in general provided by pharmacies, who receive a fee per prescribed item. About 10% of GPs provide pharmaceuticals to their own patients. They receive an additional capitation fee for each publicly insured patient on their list. Since January 1st 1992, expenditures for prescribed drugs have been added to the AWBZ scheme.

One of the major problems of cost containment has been that the government could control capacity, prices and tariffs, but not the volume of production. In fact, the financing of the individual suppliers by *per diem* rates could be called an output-oriented, open-ended budget system. This situation ended in 1983, when a 'prospective' budget system (a fixed amount per institution, allocated in advance) was introduced for all the organizations offering intramural health care. Because the new payment system was also intended as an incentive to improve efficiency, it was determined that, if a hospital spent less than its budget, it could add the surplus to its reserves. On the other hand, if expenditures exceeded a hospital's budget limit, it was financially responsible for that deficit (Maarse et al 1992). This new financing system has been effective in controlling costs, the growth rate fell from about 13% in the 1974-1982 period to about 2.4% in 1983-1985.

It should be clear that the incentives of the prospective fixed budget system differ radically from the earlier output-oriented open-ended payment system with *per diem* rates, because in the old system hospitals had a strategic interest in a high level of production. At first this budget system was based on historical costs, but it has gradually developed into a more advanced budget formula, which means that efficiency differences between hospitals no longer have any influence on the budget level. The budget is determined by capacity variables such as the number of inhabitants in the catchment area, the number of beds, numbers of specialists (in Full Time Equivalents) and production variables such as the number of admissions, nursing days etc. (Table 2). Additional agreements are required for some specific high-cost treatments such as cardiac surgery or renal dialysis.

This new remuneration system gives hospital management greater freedom to make their own decisions. Hospitals have become more autonomous, they are allowed to realise 'profits', and the hospital management can benefit if it is able to improve efficiency and reduce costs. In short a more market-like behaviour is expected from the hospitals.

Table 2. Survey of variables determining hospital budgets

Budget parameters	Remuneration in Dutch Guilders	% of total budget
Capacity indicators:		
No. of authorized beds	11,000	9 %
No. of specialist units	335,000	25 %
Availability indicator:		
No. of persons in catchment area	80	15 %
Production volume indicators:		
No. of inpatient days	60	12 %
No. of admissions	1,150	20 %
No. of nursing days	410	2 %
No. of first visits to outpatient departments	150	14 %

Towards a more market-oriented approach

The Dutch government is planning a radical reform of the whole health care system. The key features of the proposed system are: the introduction of a compulsory health insurance system covering all citizens, abolition of the privileges of the Sickness Funds in carrying out the public insurance programme, and abolition of price regulation (OECD 1992). Greater competition between the insurers and the suppliers is expected to ensure efficiency. Social efficiency should be controlled by public choices about the services which are covered by public health insurance. It is intended to increase consumption efficiency by introducing deductibles and co-payments. The reforms should be completed in 1995.

The key features of the proposed system centre on the gradual introduction of compulsory health insurance covering all citizens and including 95% of the current public insurance package. Services such as physiotherapy, birth control, and some dental services may not be included. However no decisions have yet been made on this question. The public insurance scheme will be 85% financed by an income-related premium (e.g. percentage-of-income) and 15% by a fixed premium. The income-related premium will be collected by the tax department and paid to a Central Fund, from where it will be distributed among the insurers on a specially weighted basis. The insured will pay the fixed premium directly to the insurers.

The amount of the fixed premium will vary with the number of insured persons in a family and the amount of any deductibles. The Sickness Funds will no longer have a privileged position in the public insurance programme: commercial insurers will also be involved. In fact, all insurers will be required to offer the basic package and accept any applicant. This compulsory acceptance should avoid the problem of some insurers refusing high risks. The insurers are expected to compete on the basis of the fixed part of the premium for the public insurance scheme and the premiums of the private supplementary insurance schemes. These changes in the insurance market can be expected to have a significant influence on the relations between insurers and health services organizations. The latter are no longer protected by regulated prices or contractual obligations, so insurers are expected to have more market power in buying services from the providers. This is expected to produce the right incentives to provide services according to demand and to shift resources where required. Readiness to shift resources is expected to be improved by competitive forces in the suppliers' market, in which hospitals play a dominant role.

THEORY, METHODS AND DATA SOURCES

Porter (1980, 1988) offers a model of the structure of the external environment which can be utilised to analyse the extent to which conditions exist for competition. This model covers the main variables which influence the competitive force on an industry. His approach is based on the view that competitive forces are determined not only by rivalry between suppliers on the same market, but also by certain characteristics of the market structure. These characteristics are: the bargaining power of suppliers and buyers, the threat of new entrants and the threat from substitutes. These market characteristics, applied to the market for hospital services, are represented in figure 1.

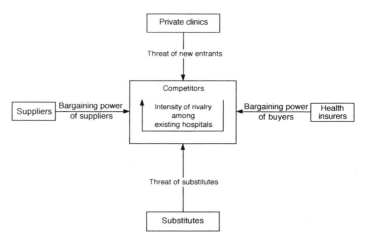

Figure 1. Model of competitive forces (Porter 1988)

This analysis will first address the rivalry between hospitals; and then analyze the bargaining power of the health insurers; and finally the threat of new entrants, especially at the position of private clinics, a relatively new phenomena in the Netherlands, as, until recently, the establishment and operation of hospital services was very strongly regulated.

For the empirical part of this study data from the Dutch Hospital Institute has been utilised. Data about health insurers was gathered in part through a questionnaire sent to all health insurers in the Netherlands, and a follow-up by telephone. Data about private clinics were collected by telephone interviews.

EMPIRICAL RESULTS

Rivalry among hospitals — an historical approach

As previously stated, rivalry between hospitals is one of the five forces that determines competition in the industry. The intensity of rivalry is determined by a number of factors:

- The market structure in terms of the number of competitors in the market and their market shares. If there are only a small number of hospitals in the market, or if one has a dominant position, it is probable that rivalry will be lower than if there are many hospitals or they are roughly equal in size and power.
- Industry growth. If growth is slow or absent, hospitals that wish to grow will probably need to take over the market share of competitors.
- Excess capacity. Is there is substantial excess capacity, rivalry should be greater.
- The level of differentiation costs. If switching cost are low, it is relatively easy for buyers to change suppliers, and therefore rivalry tends to be higher.
- If fixed costs are high this creates a strong temptation to cut prices.
- Exit barriers. If exit costs are high, exit will be a less attractive alternative when profitability is under pressure. In such a situation rivalry tends to increase.

Table 3. Concentration indices of the hospital market in 27 Dutch health regions (C_1 & C_2)

		1978	1990	Qualification
C_1 regions	$C_1 < 25\%$	13	4	moderate market power
	$25\% < C_1 < 50\%$	11	19	significant market power
	$50\% < C_1 < 75\%$	2	2	great market power
	$C_1 < 25\%$	1	2	monopolistic market power
C_2 regions	$C_2 < 50\%$	16	6	moderate market power
	$50\% < C_2 < 75\%$	7	16	substantial market power
	$C_2 > 75\%$	4	5	strong market power

So as to evaluate whether changes in the market structure of hospital services contribute to rivalry or not, an examination of the changes in the structure of the hospital market is necessary, for this purpose 1992 is compared with 1978. Use is made of concentration indices.[2] Table 3 shows the values of the concentration

---

[2]   The degree of concentration measures the market shares of the x largest enterprises and is formulated as:

$$C = \sum_{i=1}^{x} Mi\,(i = 1..x, x+1...n)^2$$

Mi is the market share of the ith enterprise and Mi > 0. The value for i is usually 1, giving C_1, the market concentration of the market leader, but values of 2 and 4 are also used, to give the concentration index of the two or four biggest enterprises, C_2 and C_4

index for 1978 and 1990, computed on the basis of the numbers of hospital beds in use per health region. In the Netherlands there are 27 health regions, which can be considered as local markets.

Sheperd (1985) suggested a number of criteria which can be used to categorise the relations among competitors. If the market leader is not threatened by a competitor and his market share is more than 50%, the leading hospital has substantial market power, enough to dominate the local market. If the market share of the four biggest hospitals (C_4) is between 60% and 100%, the market can be characterised as oligopolistic. Goos (1989) categorizes a market with a C_4 between 25% and 50% as a moderately concentrated market. A market with less than 50 competitors none of which have a market share of more than 10%, can be characterised as monopolistic competition. Only if there are more than 50 competitors with small market shares does the market reflect perfect competition or, in Porter's (1980) terms, there is effective competition. The data in table 3 shows that in 1978, 14 out of 27 health regions had a C_1 greater than 25%, and 3 had a C_1 greater than 50%. In 1990 there were 23 health regions with a C_1 greater or equal to 25% and 4 regions had a C_1 greater or equal to 50%.

By 1990 the number of regions with a comparable C_2 had grown to 21. In both 1978 and 1990 the C_4 of all health regions was at least 40%, so it would be difficult to characterize these market structures as providing effective competition. The increasing concentration is especially caused by mergers, 61 during the period under consideration, and by the exit of 22 hospitals from the market. There were only 5 new entrants to the market, which indicates serious access limitations. In 1990 there were 163 hospitals left, compared to 240 in 1978. A merger is defined as the legal integration of one or more hospitals, including the joining of their licenses. An exit movement means that the license of a hospital has been withdraw, and therefore the hospital has moved out of the market.

The Herfindahl-Hirschman index equals the sum of the squared market shares of all competitors.[3] The advantage of this index is that it not only uses the data for the largest enterprises, but of all the enterprises in the market. If the HHI exceeds 0.18, the market is categorized as strongly concentrated (Vita and Schuman 1991). As we can see from table 4, in 1978 only 15 out of 27 health regions had a value lower than 0.18. Between 1978 and 1990 the HHI increased in most health regions. This

---

respectively. If the concentration index of the biggest company equals 1, there is a monopoly market.

[3]   The Herfindahl-Hirschman index (HHI) equals the sum of the squared market shares of the n hospitals in a given health region:

$$HHI = \sum_{i=1}^{n} (Mi)^2$$

Mi is the market share of the ith hospital, and $Mi > 0$. The HHI takes into account the relative magnitude of the market shares. Its maximum value is 1, in a monopoly situation. HHI approaches zero where there are many hospitals with equal market shares.

confirms the picture given by the concentration indices.[4] The increase in the HHI is partly caused by the decrease in the number of hospitals in the health regions and partly by increasing inequalities in the market shares of hospitals. Only one region had an HHI of 1.00 in 1990, indicating a regional monopolistic market. In 1990 only four health regions had a moderate concentration.

Table 4. Concentration of the hospital market in 27 Dutch health regions, 1978-1990 based on the Herfindahl-Hirschman index (HHI)

		1978	1990	Qualification
No. of regions	HHI < 0.18	15	4	moderate concentration
	0.18 < HHI < 0.50	10	20	substantial concentration
	0.50 < HHI	2	3	strong concentration

The intensity of rivalry between 1978 and 1990

The fluidity index (FI) can be used as another measure for rivalry among hospitals. This index[5] measures the change in the market shares of hospitals in a certain health region. Table 5 gives the values of FI for each health region.

Table 5. Fluidity index per health region, 1978-1990 (based on occupied beds)

No. of regions	< 0.25	23	moderate rivalry
	0.25 < FI < 1.00	4	significant rivalry
	FI > 1	0	strong rivalry

In none of the regions was the FI greater than 1. In 23 regions the value of the FI is even smaller than 0.25. In regions with small concentration-indices the value of the FI is as expected relatively high.

On the basis of these results we may conclude that the current structures of the local hospitals markets do not in general positively contribute to rivalry among hospitals. Between 1978 and 1991 the number of hospitals decreased in all health

---

[4] There is a significant positive correlation between HHI 1990 and the C_1, C_2 and C_4 in 1990 ($p < 0,001$).

[5] The fluidity index measures the degree of rivalry on the basis of shifts in the market shares of hospitals in a given health region. The index is defined as:

$$F = \sum_{i=1}^{n} Di$$

Di equals the difference in the market shares of the ith hospital over a given time period (between t-1, and t). Di is determined by $Di = | Mi(t) - Mi(t-1) |$. F is a minimum, at zero, where no shifts in market shares have occurred and its maximum equals 2. A situation in which F_1 is categorized as showing strong rivalry.

regions, so that concentration increased. This trend to increasing concentration is a serious threat for rivalry among hospitals (Schut *et al* 1990).

Four reasons can be given for this increase in concentration. First, since the early seventies the government has carried out a policy of regional planning of hospital capacities, which encouraged hospital mergers (Schut *et al* 1990). The planning policy was *inter alia* based on the condition that every hospital should afford at least two full time equivalents of every basic medical specialisation. An additional condition was the minimal number of beds of 175 (Schut 1989). So merger has often functioned as a last means of survival.

A second reason is the assumed advantages of scale (Schut 1989). Big hospitals are assumed to have advantages of scale although there is little empirical evidence for this. The presence of a specific medical specialisation, which coincides mostly with the magnitude of hospitals, is more likely to be a determinant of the cost structure (Aert 1977). This result is confirmed by hospital directors after a merger has taken place (Schut *et al* 1990).

A third motive for merging is the desire of hospital managements to be able to deliver better quality health services. The bigger the hospital the more types of medical specialisation could be offered, the more investments in expensive and advanced technologies and the better the capability to follow the trend for sub-specialisations and super specialisations (Ministry 1992).

The fourth positive factor is related to the remuneration system for hospitals. This system is marked by a positive relation between the number of different types of medical specialists who are part of the hospital and the value of some of the budget parameters. The number of medical specialists is *inter alia* limited by the number of people living in the service area. Therefore merging is an adequate instrument for increasing the budget per inhabitant (Ministry 1986).

Thus, government regulation contributes to the increasing concentration of hospitals. This change could be expected to reduce rivalry and competition. This is one of the central issues of the health care reform mentioned previously. At the end of 1992 the Minister of Health was reticent to consent to intended mergers (Ministry 1992). Only small hospitals (less than 200 beds) will be able to merge unhindered.

Bargaining power of hospital care buyers

Health insurers can be considered the most important buyers of hospital care. Porter (1980) suggested seven factors which determine the buyers' bargaining power. A buyer group is powerful if:

- It is concentrated or purchases in large volume.
- The products it purchases represent a significant fraction of its suppliers' costs.
- The products it purchases from the industry are standard or undifferentiated.
- Switching costs are small.

- It earns low profits, which creates added incentive to lower its purchasing costs.
- The buyers pose a credible threat of integrating backward to make the industry's product.
- Price sensitivity will be greater when the industry's product is unimportant to the quality of the buyers' products or services.
- Buyers are well informed about cost structures.

Degree of concentration of the health insurance market

The concentration of health insurers in each health region was measured, and compared with the concentration indices of the hospital market. Table 6 shows the value of various concentration indices for health insurers.

Table 6. Concentration indices of the health insurance market (Spring 1992)

		C_1	C_2	C_4	HHI
No. of regions	index < 25%	-	-	-	10
	25% < index < 50%	18	3	-	16
	50% < index < 75%	9	17	14	1
	index > 75%	-	7	13	-

From these figures it can be concluded that the health insurers' market is substantially, if not strongly concentrated in most regional health markets. In 9 regions, the biggest health insurer has a market share of at least 50% and in all other regions this is at least 25%. If we look at the C_2 index, it appears that in 24 health regions, the two biggest health insurers have an market share of at least 50%. Using the C_4 index, this level of concentration is reached in all regions. Finally the HHI index indicates substantially unequal market shares. This high level of concentration in the health insurance market is to a great extent caused by the territorial division of markets by the Sickness Funds (table 7).

Comparison of the CIs of the regional insurers markets with the CIs of the regional hospital markets enables the following observations:

- Comparison of the C_1 and the C_2 indices for the two markets shows that in the majority of regions insurers have better bargaining positions.

Table 7. Comparison of concentration indices (CI) of the hospitals and
the insurers per health region (Spring 1992)

	Hospitals CI higher	Insurers CI higher	Total no. of regions
C_1	7	20	27
C_2	11	16	27
C_4	23	4	27
HHI	13	14	27

- The opposite applies to the C_4 index as an indicator of relative market power.
  In this case, hospitals have relatively stronger market power in the majority of
  regions. This is because, until recently, Sickness Funds had divided the markets
  territorially. These Sickness Funds have in general a market share of about
  65%. (Hartog and Janssen 1992b).

If we look at the map of the Netherlands, it appears that, regardless of the
concentration index used, the insurers in the northern part of the country and in the
densely populated west (the so called 'Randstad') have more market power than the
hospitals.

To what extent do the products insurers purchase represent a significant fraction of their costs?

The extent to which an insurer is sensitive to prices depends on the proportion of
the total costs of the insurer which are accounted for by hospital costs, and on the
type of insurer. It is possible to distinguish three types of private health insurance
companies: commercial insurers, mutual non-profit insurance companies, and
Sickness Fund related non-profit insurers. Most of the commercial insurers offer the
whole range of insurance products. This contrasts with the mutual non-profit
insurers, who generally offer only health insurance. The same holds for the Sickness
Fund related non-profit insurers, although recently some of the latter are extending
the range of insurance schemes they offer. The Sickness Funds are specialized in
health insurance schemes. Until 1993, the tariffs of most health care services were
regulated by government. Although this regulation is changing to maximum tariffs,
there is still almost no price competition to be observed.

The products it purchases from the industry are standard or undifferentiated

The basic services that are offered by different hospitals can be characterized as
homogeneous. However there is differentiation in the area of highly specialized
services which are not everywhere on offer. Because academic hospitals, which
incorporate a medical school, are allowed to deliver the same services for higher
prices, insurers might wish to switch to the non-academic general hospitals.
However, thus far there have been no known examples of such a switch.

Extent of switching costs.

The switching costs for insurers are mainly administrative costs, plus the risk of loosing some customers who are willing to switch insurance companies in order to keep their relationship with a certain doctor or hospital. It may be expected that this risk factor be more important than administrative costs.

Staten (1987) mentioned two factors that may generate substantial switching costs for the insurer. Firstly,the patient is influenced by the GP making the referral, who would be expected to consider quality aspects rather than costs. Therefore, if the GP wants to refer a patient to a hospital which has no contract with a certain insurer, the patient could decide to switch to another insurance company which is in business with that hospital. Staten (1987) also observed that patients put a high value on travel time and that they try to minimize travel costs (see also Janssen 1992). So patients will in general, *ceteris paribus,* not switch easily to another hospital. Staten concludes that a patient in such a situation is more willing to switch insurance companies. An insurer has to take these switching costs into account when considering ending a contract with a hospital.

Profitability and reserves of buyers

Sickness Funds have not until now had any financial reserves, which makes the prices of health services very important to them. Private commercial insurers are able to take more risks, depending on the magnitude of their financial reserves. After the health care reforms, these insurers will be permitted to pay higher prices, in contrast to the Sickness Funds. For the same reason hospitals are in a relatively stronger position, *ceteris paribus,* if a Sickness Fund is on the other side of the bargaining table.

Threat of backward integration by buyers

Backward integration by health insurers has rarely occurred in the Netherlands. There are only a few insurers who operate dental centres or maternity departments. In fact, legislation forbids Sickness Funds operating health care services, although this restriction will be abolished under the proposed health care reform (Tweede Kamer 1990).

Organizations such as the American Health Maintenance Organizations do not appear in the Netherlands. Recently some initiatives have been taken in the field of buying medical materials such as disposables so as to offer these directly to the insured. Additionally this far, there is no apparent threat of forward integration by hospitals.

Quality is more important than price

Quality is one of the most important features of medical services and a large part of the regulations are focused on this issue. The referring GP will also take quality into account. Quality has in the past not been expressed in the level of tariffs, but if there is further deregulation, as is intended, it is expected that quality and price will be more related to each other. Therefore the bargaining power of insurers will be strengthened. Hospitals will be forced to show how prices and tariffs are related to quality.

Knowledge of buyers.

Bargaining power is also determined by the extent to which insurers have accurate information about the hospitals offering services. At present, the problem is that insurers have a great deal of data about the way their customers have been medically treated, but they are not really able to transform this data into information that could be used in the bargaining process. Therefore the aggregation of data by types of specialists or diagnosis groups is needed. This process has just commenced.

Conclusions about the bargaining power of health insurers

Using Porter's model (1980) as an analytical tool to consider the bargaining power of health insurers, the following conclusions can be drawn:

i.   In those regions where hospitals have monopolistic supplier positions, these hospitals have great bargaining power than the health insurers.
ii. Sickness Funds have, for the time being, a larger market share than commercial insurers, so that their bargaining power is also greater. On the other hand Sickness Funds have a smaller product range than the commercial general insurers, and less financial reserves. So they are forced to achieve good results in the bargaining process. Until 1993, hospitals were protected by tariff regulation. We may expect that the bargaining process will become more fluid in the future.
iii. The services of the hospitals are marked by a certain degree of differentiation and by the great value that is given to the quality of the services. Still, price is a minor element in the bargaining process, although it is expected that further deregulation will increase price sensitivity, especially for the Sickness Funds.
iv. Patients are emotionally connected to physicians and hospitals. This contributes to the bargaining power of the hospitals. Insurers are in a relatively stronger position when contracting with hospitals operating in areas which are densely populated.
v.   Until now backward integration has been a marginal phenomenon, due in part to restrictive regulation. In the near future no significant threat is expected from insurers. In general health insurers, as buyers, have little insight into the real cost structure of the services they buy.

In short, the bargaining power of hospitals in relation to the insurers is still very strong (see table 8). The intended health care reforms will shift the power balance

Table 8. Survey of bargaining power of insurers on the basis of
determining factors of Porter (1988)

Determining factor	Bargaining power of health insurers	Strongest bargaining position
Concentration	In 20 health regions the C_1 of insurers is greater than that of hospitals. In 16 health regions the C_2 of insurers is greater than that of hospitals. In 4 health regions the C_4 of insurers is greater than that of hospitals. In 14 health regions the HHI of insurers is greater than that of hospitals	$+ / -$
Product mix buyer	About 67% of the market is served by mono-product insurers (Sickness Funds). The remaining insurers are more or less multi-product suppliers. However price sensitivity was diminished by tariff regulation until recently	Hospitals
Product differentiation	Degree of homogeneity of health care services is very low	Hospitals
Switching costs	Switching costs for the insurers are significant, especially in less densely populated areas	Hospitals
Profits/reserves of buyers	About 67% of the insurers have some financial reserves. Until recently tariff regulation diminished price sensitivity	Hospitals
Backward integration	No backward integration by insurers , nor threat of this	Hospitals
Quality health care services	Quality of health care services is important, price sensitivity is less important	Hospitals
Information	In general buyers have only general data on hospitals. Bargaining power depends on the ability to transform this data into useful information	$+ / -$

to the advantage of the insurers, but the hospitals are still expected to have a relatively strong bargaining position.

Threat of new entrants: private clinics

The presence of potential new entrants to a market is one of the factors that determines the level of competitive power. The private commercial clinics can be considered as new entrants to the hospital services market (Den Hartog and Janssen, 1992c).

There has been strong growth in the number of private clinics in the Netherlands over time. At the moment there are 44 clinics in the Netherlands, in which 120 physicians are working. Most of these private clinics are located in the western, densely-populated part of the Netherlands. There are only 8 health regions, out of 27, in which no private clinics are located.

Seven clinics offer more than one specialisation. As an indication of capacity, twenty-four clinics have at least one operating theatre. Clinics without operating theatres in general specialise in dermatology (7), phlebology (5), fertility treatment (4) and ophthalmology (2). Two ophthalmological clinics use laser techniques.

Other studies have shown that the establishment of clinics is determined by factors such as the ratio of outpatient treatment to clinical treatment, the degree of dependence on other types of specialists, the length of waiting lists, and the density of population. All these factors contribute positively to the establishment of private clinics. However most of the physicians working in a private clinic are also connected to a hospital (Den Hartog and Janssen 1992c).

Hospitals have almost no formal opportunities to prevent the establishment of private clinics. Until 1993, hospitals were not allowed to operate independent price policies because of the tariff regulation. This is in contrast to the private clinics who function outside the legislation. Almost half of the Sickness Funds do no business with these clinics because of their more or less illegal status. All private commercial insurers do business with these clinics (Zwetsloot and Janssen 1993).

It is too soon to consider the current number of private clinics as a serious threat to the hospitals. The specialists' opportunities to switch their practice from the hospital to an independent clinic are limited for technical and financial reasons. However the very existence of these clinics function as an eye-opener for the hospitals. As a result many hospitals have undertaken activities to meet the preferences of their customers better. Data systems have been improved, waiting rooms have been painted, etc. Some hospitals are starting private clinics by themselves to offer small-scale, customer-friendly, services.

Structure of the hospital services market — some conclusions

It can be seen that the environment of hospitals is significantly changing. These changes can, in a certain way, be characterized as paradoxical. A more concentrated market, that is to say with less decision centres, which leads to less uncertainty for the participants can be observed. Conversely, there is increasing uncertainty, caused by the following factors:

- Liberalization of tariff regulation causes more uncertainty in their relationship with the insurers. This is in conformity with one of the government's goals with regard to the health care reforms.
- Until 1989, the government offered guarantees for financial loans. Since the government has ended this role, banks and other financial institutions, which extend loans to hospitals, have become more influential. They set conditions, such as the elimination of over-capacity, and they screen the quality of management of hospitals.
- Liberalization of the regulations on the establishment of physicians and clinics gives rise to the threat of new entrants. The growing numbers of private clinics being established is an expression of this threat.

- Patients are freer in that they are better informed, critical consumers. Although the meaning of this change is limited in a monopolistic market, hospitals have to take account of this.
- When the health care reforms are introduced, the importance of collective contracts between employers and health insurers will increase. The situation will be more like that in the United States, were 80% of insurance schemes are part of collective contracts.

In summation, it can be concluded that the uncertainty with regard to the environment of hospitals has grown, and that there is more need to formulate strategies.

CONSEQUENCES FOR STRATEGIC MANAGEMENT

Strategy, or strategic management can be defined as a coherent unity of vision and behaviour, focused on the maintenance and if possible improvement of vitality and the position of an organization in its environment (Meijer 1990). A strategy is based on interaction between the goals of an organization, its environment and the features of its internal organization. Or as Porter (1988) states: "The essence of strategy formulation is coping with competition".

The key to growth is to stake out a position that is less vulnerable to competing hospitals and less vulnerable to erosion by buyers, suppliers, and substitute goods. Establishing such a position can take many forms: solidifying relationships with good customers, differentiating the product, integrating backward or forward, or establishing technological leadership (Porter 1988). Porter distinguishes 3 kinds of competitive strategies: (1) cost leadership (2) differentiation and (3) focus. These categories have been used in research into health care markets. Whitehead *et al* (1989) used these categories to analyze the strategic management of Health Maintenance Organizations (HMOs) in the US, and Winter and Den Hartog (1992) and Winter and Van Merode (1993) used the same categories to analyze the strategic management of hospitals in the Netherlands.

Miles and Snow (1978) provide a typology of possible reactions to changes in the market. They distinguished defenders, prospectors, analyzers and reactors. Shortell (1990) applied these categories to American hospitals. He also felt that a majority (55.2%) of the hospitals could be categorized as analyzers, 23.8% as prospectors, 24.5% as reactors and only 6.5% as defenders. They also concluded that the number of analyzers was reducing, while the number of prospectors was increasing. The number of defenders and reactors remained more or less stable. Preliminary results of research in the Netherlands (Den Hartog and Winter 1992) indicate that this typology is applicable to the strategic management of Dutch hospitals.

The Working group on Future Scenario's in Health Care (STG 1990) in its report, called "The hospital in the 21st century", presented two possible scenarios, namely a disengagement scenario and a network scenario. In the first scenario specialists work increasingly in private clinics. This is as a reaction to the large-scale standardized hospitals. The state will withdraw, which will be expressed in deregulation and reduction of the cover of compulsory health insurance. It is also expected that medical technology will in future be applicable on a smaller local scale and that the prices of advanced techniques will fall significantly.

In the network scenario, hospitals are the dominant supply centres for health care services. It is expected that regional networks will develop, in which hospitals complement each other. All hospitals will have the basic functions, more advanced functions will be regionally concentrated and some very advanced specialisations will be organized on a supra-regional scale. Within the organization a process of deconcentration will start, for example in the form of satellite outdoor treatment centres. In this scenario the state continues to play a significant role in the regulation of access and quality and controlling expenditures and tariffs.

In a recently published report of the Ministry (1990) it is speculated that in the future, hospital functions may be reduced to "cures" and that the "care" function will take place outside the hospital.

It can be expected that the process of concentration will continue, despite the more restrictive attitude announced by the Minister of Health regarding mergers. Also that despite the intended reduction in government regulation, the tradition of self-regulation will remain a significant feature of the health care market. On the basis of the dynamic market theory of De Jong (1989), the final section of this paper explores four possible changes in the health care market.

Backward integration by insurers

Backward integration by insurers means that insurers go into the business of supplying health care. There are some initiatives in the Netherlands, which look like the American HMOs. However, in the Netherlands insurers do not have any tradition of activities outside the insurance industry itself. Such a move could be more attractive to the one-product health insurers. At the moment the latter are attractive partners for general insurance companies, since the health care reforms will deregulate statutory health insurance. Moreover, there is a trend towards mergers between insurance companies and banks, which will result in great multi-product financial organisations. Therefore we may conclude that backward integration by insurers is less likely to be a dominant trend in the near future.

Forward integration by hospitals

Forward integration means that health care suppliers move into the insurance business. Considering the dominant trends in the insurance sector it would seem very unlikely that suppliers would be able to enter the insurance market. The move towards collective contracting with employers also gives the multi-product insurers a lot of advantages.

Diversification by hospitals

Diversification by hospitals refers to the network scenario mentioned above. In this scenario hospitals work together with GPs, health centres, home nursing organizations etc.. In fact this is a strategy for which some hospitals in the Netherlands are explicitly striving. It is clear that the traditional health professionals working out of hospitals feel this change as a threat to their independence. However if hospitals succeed in offering complete service packages, this could be very attractive to the buyers, namely the insurers and the consumers.

Specialisation or vertical dis-integration by hospitals

Specialisation or vertical dis-integration means that traditional hospital services are offered by separate, independent organizations. This could include private clinics, maternity homes and hospices for the dying. Such a movement resembles the disengagement scenario, mentioned above.

CONCLUSIONS

On the basis of this analysis of the features and changes in the Dutch health care market it is concluded that the health care system in the Netherlands is in transition from being a subsystem of the public sector to an industry ruled by the same basic rules as all other industries. Price negotiations are becoming part of the bargaining process between suppliers and insurers. The financial risks of organizations and uncertainty in general are growing, demanding a more entrepreneurial attitude. Because of the strong concentration process it is very doubtful that rivalry and competition are growing. However other changes in the environment of hospitals will force them to pay more attention to explicit strategic management. The challenge to the government is to keep realising public goals with the help of a privatised health care and health insurance industry (Janssen and Van der Made 1990).

Porter's model has proved to be a very helpful tool in understanding long-term developments in the structure of the health care industry. The application of research in the tradition of "the theory of industrial organizations" to the health care sector should be stimulated, not only for scientific purposes but also to gain a better understanding of adequate entrepreneurship in a health care market working for public goals.

REFERENCES

Aert, J.H. (1977), Ziekenhuiskosten in econometrisch perspectief, Utrecht.

Centraal Bureau van de Statistiek (1991), Statistisch Jaarboek, Voorburg.

Doel, J. van den (1981), 'Begrip en meting van economische macht', Roos, W.A.A.M. de (ed.), De pluriforme economische macht, Alphen a.d. Rijn, 13 - 55.

Financieel overzicht zorg, various volumes, Staats Uitgeverij, The Hague.

Goos, a.,(1989) 'Koncentratie verzekerd?', Tijdschrift voor politieke economie, 12, 52-73.

Groenewegen, R., Van der Zee, J. and Van Haaften, R., (1991), Remunerating General Practitioners in Western Europe, Avebury, Aldershot.

Grünwald, C.A., (1987) Beheersing van de gezondheidszorg (thesis), Utrecht.

Hartog, M. den, and R.T.J.M. Janssen, (1992a), Vraag en aanbod in de Nederlandse Gezondheidszorg, Department of Health Economics, Maastricht.

Hartog, M. den, and R.T.J.M. Janssen, (1992b), Concurrentie en rivaliteit tussen ziekenhuizen, Department of Health Economics, Maastricht.

Hartog, M. den, and R.T.J.M. Janssen,(1992c), Privé-klinieken nader onderzocht, Department of Health Economics, Maastricht.

Hartog, M. den, and J. Winter, (1992) Strategisch management in Nederlandse ziekenhuizen, Department of Health Economics, Maastricht.

Janssen, Richard, (1992), Time Prices on the Demand for GP Services, Social Science and Medicine, vol. 34, No 7, pp. 725-733.

Janssen, Richard and Jan van der Made,(1990), 'Privatisation in Health Care: Concepts, motives and policies', Health Policy, nr 14,1990, pp 191-202.

Janssen, Richard and Jan van der Made, (1991), Privatisation in Western European health care: A comparative study. International Journal of Health Sciences vol. 2, no. 2, 63 - 83.

Jong, H.W. de (1989), Dynamische Markttheorie, Stenfert Kroese, Leiden.

Maarse, J.A.M., A. van der Horst and E.J.E. Molin, (1992), Hospital budgeting in the Netherlands: Effects on Hospital Services, Maastricht.

Miles, R.E. and C.C. Snow, (1978), Organizational strategy, structure and process, New York.

Miller and Friesen, (1984), Organizations: a quantum view, New Jersey.

Ministry of Health, (1986), Richtlijnen Wet Ziekenhuisvoorzienigen, The Hague.

Ministry of Health, (1987), Bereidheid tot verandering, The Hague.

Ministry of Health, (1988), Change Assured, The Hague, 1988.

Ministry of Health, (1992), Positionering van ziekenhuiszorg, The Hague.

Meijer, A.W.M., (1990), Instellingen en strategisch beleid, Maarse, J. and I. Mur (eds), Beleid en Beheer in de Gezondheidszorg, Assen, 312 - 336.

OECD, (1992), The reform of health care, A comparative Analysis of Seven OECD Countries, Paris.

Porter, M.E. (1980), Competitive Strategy, Free Press, New York.

Porter, M.E., (1988), Strategy Analysis, Quin, J.B., H. Mintzberg, and R.M. James (eds), The strategy process, concepts, contexts and cases, Prentice Hall International, 57 - 70

Schut, F.T., (1989), Mededingingsbeleid in de gezondheidszorg, De Tijdstroom, Lochem.

Schut, F.T., W. Greenberg, and W.P.M.M. van de Ven, (1990), Antitrust policy in the Dutch health care; Relevance of EEC competition policy and US Antitrust Practice, Erasmus University, Rotterdam.

Sheperd, W.G., (1985), The economics of industrial organizations, Prentice Hall, New Jersey.

Shortell, S.M., (1990), Choices for American Hospitals, Yossey Bas, San Francisco.

Staten, M., (1987), 'Marketshare and the illusion of power', Journal of Health Economics, 6, 43 - 56.

Stuurgroep Toekomstscenario's Gezondheidszorg, (STG, 1990), Het ziekenhuis in de 21e eeuw, een aanzet tot discussie, Utrecht.

Stuurgroep Toekomstscenario's Gezondheidszorg, (STG, 1992), Toekomstscenario's voor eerstelijnszorg en thuiszorg, Houten.

Tweede Kamer, (1990), vergaderjaar 1990-1991, 21592, nr. 3, Memorie van Toelichting, The Hague.

Vita M.G., and L. Schumann, (1991), 'The competitive effects of horizontal mergers in the hospital industry: a closer look', Journal of Health Economics, 10, 359-372.

Whitehead, C.J., J.D. Blair, R.R. Smith, T.W. Nix and G.T. Savage, (1989), 'Stakeholder supportiveness and strategic vulnerability: Implications for competitive strategy in the HMO industry', Health Care Management Review, 14(3), 65 - 76.

Zwetsloot M.M.J., and R.T.J.M. Janssen (1993), 'Partikuliere klinieken en ziektekostenverzekeraars', Medisch Contact, (48) 2, 39 - 41.

19 Factors Affecting Physician Efficiency in Managing Hospitalized Patients

LAWTON R. BURNS[1], JON A. CHILINGERIAN[2] & DOUGLAS R. WHOLEY[3]

[1]*University of Arizona, U.S.A.*
[2]*Brandeis University, U.S.A.*
[3]*Carnegie Mellon University, U.S.A.*

INTRODUCTION

There is a great deal of interest in studying variations in health care utilization in the United States. Variations in utilization patterns are the central concern of three major movements: the trend to develop clinical practice guidelines for physicians (partially supported by the federally-sponsored Medical Treatment Effectiveness Program), increased research on the effect of practice patterns on patient outcomes (also federally-supported through the Agency for Health Care Policy Research), and the trend to institutionalize continuous quality improvement (or total quality management) methods in health care organizations.

One reason for the great interest in understanding variations is the belief that more standardized utilization patterns (i.e., narrow range of variation) result in higher quality and lower cost. This belief has spawned a number of hospital strategies aimed at cost control, such as increased utilization review procedures and practice profiles of physicians. Some research suggests that the growth in hospital expenditures over time is largely due to the increased intensity of resource use per admission, rather than the increased number of admissions (Freeland and Schendler 1983).

These federal efforts concerning practice guidelines and the hospital strategies presume that physicians are largely responsible for the increased intensity of services provided and the variability in resources utilized. There is considerable debate and related research on the locus of control over hospital and healthcare spending, however. The work of Wennberg and his colleagues (Wennberg and Gittelsohn 1975; Wennberg, Barnes, and Zubkoff 1982) suggests that physicians exhibit their own particular styles of practice (or medical "signatures"), reflecting clinical responses to uncertainty or economic adaptations of convenience and habit. A

Strategic Issues in Health Care Management. Edited by M. Malek, J. Rasquinha and P. Vacani
© 1993 John Wiley & Sons Ltd

related theoretical paradigm argues that physicians act as self-interested income maximizers in their utilization of hospital services (Pauly and Redisch 1973; Feldstein 1988; Eisenberg 1986). Others argue that physicians increasingly must act under constraints imposed by more assertive and better-informed patients as well as the dictates of the patient's health plan (e.g., utilization and financial controls wielded by managed care firms). Finally, there is some question whether observed variations in resource use reflect the imprecision in current patient classification systems. The question here is whether different physicians treat similar patients differently, or do classification systems lump together different types of patients treated by the same physician?

The present paper seeks to address these issues by examining the contribution of physician factors to the explanation of variability in hospital inpatient resource utilization. Following prior research (Johnson, Dowd, Morris, and Lurie 1989) inpatient resource use is considered here as one possible measure of the physician's practice style. The particular resource utilization measure employed here is the hospital charge per admission adjusted for the mean charge of all admissions in that particular hospital with that diagnosis in that year. Such an adjustment allows the researcher to examine the efficiency of physician practice with respect to hospital norms. The analyses seek to control for patient classification by using the patient's diagnosis related group (DRG), severity-of-illness, and specific information on secondary diagnoses and procedures. The analyses also seek to control for the contribution of other factors known to be associated with inpatient cost (e.g., patient factors, hospital factors, and region).

PRIOR RESEARCH AND HYPOTHESES

Sources of Variation in Hospital Resource Use

Over the past ten years, researchers have devoted considerable attention to the factors explaining variation in hospital resource utilization. Utilization has been measured in terms of adjusted hospital charges, length of stay, and intensity of services (e.g., inputs per stay, costs per day). Results across the different measures of utilization are fairly consistent, given the high correlation among the utilization measures themselves (Horn, Horn, and Sharkey 1984; Burns, Wholey, and Abeln 1992). Due to this consistency, as well as the relative dearth of studies regarding physician effects, we consider studies using length of stay and intensity measures relevant for this study of adjusted hospital charges.

Studies of hospital utilization have typically estimated multivariate models that incorporate the patient's clinical diagnosis classification, characteristics of the patient's health and sociodemographic status, features of the hospital, and characteristics of the physician (Hornbrook and Goldfarb 1981; Goldfarb, Hornbrook, and Higgins 1983; Horn et al. 1984; McMahon and Newbold 1986; Cromwell, Mitchell, Calore, *et al* 1987; Feinglass, Martin, and Sen 1991). Research by Horn and colleagues (Horn and Sharkey 1983; Horn *et al* 1984; Horn, Bulkley, Sharkey, *et al* 1985) as well as by Feinglass *et al* (1991) suggests that the majority of the variation in hospital charges is accounted for by the patient's severity-of-illness and case-mix (e.g., the disease classification system). Other patient factors are also significant predictors of utilization. These include both demographic factors (such as insurance status, age, gender, and income) and illness-specific factors (such as secondary diagnoses, day of week of admission, and admission source). Hospital characteristics such as urban location, teaching status, and ownership have also been found to be associated with utilization, although the direction of the latter two effects varies by diagnosis (Goldfarb *et al* 1983; Dowd, Johnson, and Madson 1986).

Physician factors also contribute to the explained variation, although less is known about specific causal effects. This relative lack of understanding is due to the use of physician identifiers (i.e. dummy variables denoting particular practitioners), rather than physician characteristics, in most of the models estimated (Horn *et al* 1984; McMahon and Newbold 1986; Feinglass *et al* 1992). Identifiers are typically used because the number of physicians in the sample is small or personal characteristics of the physician are not known. Most studies of hospital utilization lack information on the patient's physician. Some recent evidence suggests that physician factors may be a more powerful determinant of efficient utilization than hospital factors (Burns and Wholey 1991).

Hypothesis 1:   As a whole, physician factors explain a significant amount of the variation in hospital utilization.

Physician Practice Style

Several studies in the general medical economics literature examine physician influences on the cost and utilization of medical care (Eisenberg 1986). These influences have been described in terms of "surgical signatures" (Wennberg and Gittelsohn 1982) and "practice styles" (Eisenberg 1986). The studies that specify physician effects focus on background characteristics, practice setting, and characteristics of the physician's hospital practice. The effects of these factors have been previously described as elements of an economic model of physician behaviour, variously labelled the 'self-fulfilling practitioner' model (Eisenberg 1986) or the 'income-maximizing economic agent' model (Pauly and Redisch 1973; Feldstein 1988). These models are partly encompassed in a more recent model of the physician as the manager of a temporary firm that forms and dissolves with the admission and discharge of each new patient (Chilingerian and Glavin, 1992). All of these models suggest a number of hypothesized effects of physician background, practice setting, and hospital practice characteristics on the efficient utilization of hospital services.

Background Characteristics

Studies report that physicians' personal characteristics are associated with rates of hospitalization, length of stay, and use of diagnostic tests (Eisenberg and Nicklin 1981; Roos, Flowerdew, Wajda *et al* 1986). Younger and less experienced physicians typically utilize more hospital services, such as X-Ray exams, diagnostic tests, and intensive care (Childs and Hunter 1972; Eisenberg, 1986). Presumably, a significant portion of this higher utilization reflects inappropriate care due to immature clinical judgement. Indeed, years of experience, which is strongly correlated with age, bears the same relationship with utilization. Comparative studies of seasoned physicians and medical students report that the former are better able to recall more critical clinical cues and to differentiate relevant from irrelevant information (Coughlin and Patel 1987). Other studies have found that the number of years since medical school graduation is negatively associated with ancillary utilization (Eisenberg and Nicklin 1981).

Hypothesis 2:   Physician experience is negatively associated with the utilization of hospital services.

Specialization of practice also influences physician behaviour. The medical literature suggests that specialists provide more intensive care than do generalists (Eisenberg 1986). For example, paediatricians order more diagnostic tests than do general practitioners (Fishbane and Starfield 1981). Similarly, sub specialists order more services than do internists (Manu and Schwartz 1983). Eisenberg (1986) suggests that these differential patterns of utilization are acquired early on in the physician's residency training.

Hypothesis 3:   General practitioners are likely to utilize fewer hospital services than specialists

Hypothesis 4:   Board-certified physicians are likely to utilize more hospital services than non-board certified physicians.

Several authors have described the importance of medical school and residency training in the socialization of physicians (Bosk 1979; Fox 1988). There is some evidence that the particular medical school attended influences the physician's subsequent practice style, such as length of stay (Burns and Wholey 1991), although the causal mechanism is not well understood. Researchers have already documented the effect of foreign medical training on utilization (Roos *et al* 1986).

Hypothesis 5:   Physicians who are foreign medical graduates (FMGs) are likely to utilize more hospital services.

Hypothesis 6:   The particular medical school attended affects the physician's utilization of hospital services.

Practice Setting

Previous studies have found that characteristics of the physician's practice setting also influence practice style.   Patients in managed care settings, such as health maintenance organizations (HMOs), exhibit much lower hospital admission rates, surgical rates, ancillary use, and shorter hospital stays (Luft 1978; Newhouse, Schwartz, Williams *et al* 1985; Dowd *et al* 1986; Johnson et al 1989; Chilingerian 1989) than do patients in fee-for-service settings.   Some observers argue that prepayment arrangements found in HMOs encourage physicians to be more efficient by shifting to them part of the financial risk of treatment.

Most physicians in the U.S. do not practice exclusively in managed care (HMO) settings.   Instead, their practice consists of both fee-for-service and managed care patients.   Because physicians can not always distinguish between different payer groups without asking the patient, it is likely that they tend to treat their patients in fairly similar ways.   However, as the physician's managed care practice increases as a proportion of his/her total practice -- and thus as the physician's utilization of hospital services for these patients declines -- we suggest that physicians will tend to treat their fee-for-service patients in the same manner as the managed care patients.

Hypothesis 7:   Physicians who see a greater percentage of HMO patients in their hospital practice are likely to utilize fewer hospital services.

Hospital Practice Characteristics

There has been increasing research interest in whether the physician's volume and distribution of hospital practice influences the hospitalization experience of particular patients.   The mortality literature suggests that higher physician volume with a procedure is associated with lower mortality rates (Shortell and LoGerfor 1981; Hannan, O'Donnell, Kilburn *et al* 1989).   The major causal imputation here is that higher volume leads to better maintenance of skills, or "practice makes perfect" (Luft 1980; Flood, Scott, and Ewy 1984).   It is less clear whether increased practice volume makes the physician more efficient.   On the one hand, increased volume is associated with increased information processing needs (Galbraith 1977).   As a result, physicians may be too busy to efficiently manage their hospitalized patients. On the other hand, increased volume should lead the physician to be better versed with the procedure/illness, with the appropriate treatment regimen, and with the hospital staff, and thus be in a better position to efficiently manage the patient's hospitalization.   Higher volumes also imply capacity limits for physicians (and hospitals) that lead to shorter hospitalizations.   One prior study found that higher physician volumes are associated with shorter hospital stays for surgical patients, particularly in busy hospitals (Burns and Wholey 1991).

Hypothesis 8:   Physicians with higher volumes of patients hospitalized with the same diagnosis during the year are likely to utilize fewer services.

In addition to the volume of hospital practice, physicians vary in terms of the number and distribution of hospitals at which they practice. Some physicians practice exclusively at one facility; others practice at several hospitals and spread more of their patients among them. Elsewhere we have suggested that physicians who concentrate their practice at one hospital emphasize convenience, while those who disperse their practice to several hospitals emphasize professional autonomy (Burns, Wholey, and Huonker 1991; Wholey and Burns 1991). Given the temporal and spatial limits on the physician's ability to manage patients across a network of hospitals, we suggest that physicians who concentrate their practice and seek to maximize efficiency in their own schedule should devote greater attention to the efficient management of their patients.

Hypothesis 9:   Physicians with concentrated hospital practices should utilize fewer hospital services.

METHODS AND MEASURES

Analytic Approach

We examined the explanatory power of the physician factors in two ways. First, we assessed the contribution of the entire set of physician variables to the explained variation in adjusted hospital charges (Hypothesis 1), controlling for severity, patient, and hospital characteristics. Second, we tested hypothesized relationships between specific physician characteristics and the dependent variable (Hypotheses 2-9).

Multiple regression and analysis of covariance (ANCOVA) techniques are used to model the patient's adjusted charges as a function of severity of illness and several patient, hospital, and physician characteristics. Separate regression models are estimated for each diagnosis studied. We used the reduction in the error sum of squares to assess the significance of the contribution of physician factors as a whole to the overall explanation, and standard statistical (F-statistic) tests to assess the hypothesized relationships between the physician factors and adjusted charges.

Unit of Analysis

The unit of analysis is the individual patient seen by his/her physician in a particular hospital. This approach allows us to directly link data on the patient, physician, and hospital, thus avoiding any aggregation bias. It also allows us to examine the practice characteristics of physicians across the multiple hospitals they may utilize. In addition, the analyses are conducted separately for each of ten different diagnoses (4 medical, 4 surgical, 2 maternity). Such an approach is warranted given the differing patterns of effects across diagnoses noted by other researchers.

Patients and Conditions

The data sets (described below) used for these analyses contain information on discharges in 10 medical, surgical, and maternity DRGs. The four medical diagnoses include chronic obstructive pulmonary disease (or COPD), myocardial infarction, congestive heart failure, and a trial fibrillation. The four surgical diagnoses include coronary artery bypass without cardiac catheterization, large bowel resection, major joint procedures, and hip replacement. The two maternity conditions include caesarean section and vaginal delivery. Table 1 describes the number of discharges, mean charges, and the coefficient of variation in charges for the ten conditions.

These particular conditions were chosen on the basis of both practical and statistical grounds. For practical reasons, some of these conditions are ranked among the top twenty-five DRGs in terms of inpatient payments per capita (MEDSTAT, 1992). They thus account for a major proportion of hospital spending. Other conditions were included for statistical reasons because they possessed sufficient numbers of discharges for the analyses and exhibited some homogeneity in their treatment patterns (defined by the coefficient of variation in hospital charges). Table 1 lists the number of discharges, average hospital charges, and coefficient of variation in hospital charges for all 10 diagnoses.

Table 1. Patient characteristics and outcomes for 14 conditions selected

Medical Conditions	Number	Number of Discharges	Mean $	St. Dev $	Charges Coeff. Var.
Chronic Obstructive Pulmonary Disease	88	2,174	6,865	4,673	.68
Myocardial Infarction	121/2	5,169	11,102	6,676	.60
Congestive Heart Failure	127	8,556	6,598	4,740	.72
Atrial Fibrillation	139	1,223	3,210	2,071	.64
Surgical Conditions					
Coronary Artery Bypass	107	933	32,391	10,873	.34
Large Bowel Resection	149	634	10,424	4,492	.43
Major Joint Procedure	209	10,256	17,379	6,172	.36
Hip Fracture	211	721	9,585	4,911	.51
Maternity Conditions					
Caesarean Section	371	16,294	4,542	1,394	.31
Vaginal Delivery	373	73,752	1,893	830	.44

Dependent Variable

The dependent variable is the hospital charge for the particular patient, adjusted for the mean charge for all patients with that diagnosis treated in that hospital that year (1989 or 1990). Similar methods are employed in other studies of hospital charges (Jencks and Kay 1987; Feinglass et al. 1991). It thus reflects the deviation from the hospital norm for similar patients. Controlling for severity, positive values reflect higher than average charges and, thus, greater inefficiency in treatment; negative values reflect lower than average charges and, thus, greater efficiency.

Control Variables — Severity, Patient, and Hospital Factors

Severity of illness was measured using the Acuity Index Method (AIM) severity index developed by Iameter. This six-point scale takes into account the DRG, the primary and four secondary diagnoses, and the primary and two secondary procedures. While AIM lacks the predictive power of other severity systems, linear models using AIM provide appropriate representations of severity-utilization relationships (Thomas and Ashcraft,1991).

Several patient characteristics are included in the regression model to control for health status and demand factors affecting utilization. With regard to health status, we included dummy variables to denote the presence of specific secondary diagnoses that might affect utilization: diabetes, hypertension, anaemia, and neoplasms. In addition, we included summary measures of the number of procedures performed on the patient and the number of secondary diagnoses. We also included dummy variables denoting the source of admission (e.g., emergency room). Transfers to and from other hospitals were excluded from the analyses, as were patients with unusually long hospital stays (defined as stays exceeding the DRG trim points). Finally, we included dummy variables regarding discharge status (e.g., discharge to nursing home, discharge to other non-hospital facility) to correct for censoring in hospital stays (and thus hospital charges). Patients who died in the hospital were excluded from the analyses.

With regard to patient demand factors, we included four dummy variables denoting the patient's insurance coverage: Medicare, Medicaid/AHCCCS, commercial, and HMO/Blue Cross (self pay and other patients are the excluded contrast). We also included three dummy variables denoting admission on Friday, Saturday, and Sunday, to control for weekend admissions, and dummy variables for season due to the influx of Winter tourists to Arizona and the consequent change in hospital census and case-mix.

Several hospital characteristics were also incorporated in the regression models to control for factors associated with hospital cost. These include two dummy variables denoting investor (for-profit) ownership and public/municipal ownership (voluntary non-profit ownership is the excluded contrast), a dummy variable denoting affiliation with a residency teaching program, and four dummy variables indicating the presence of particular hospital services that might influence utilization: cardiac care unit and long-term care unit (used in the analyses of medical and surgical diagnoses), and neonatal intensive care unit and labour/delivery room (used in analyses of maternity diagnoses). We also included two dummy variables for hospital location -- one to denote rural areas, the other to denote the second largest city in the state (largest city serving as the excluded contrast) -- to control for geographic variation in utilization of services and hospital costs. Due to the small number of hospitals in the state, all of the hospital effects could be captured parsimoniously by a hospital identifier, which was used in their place.

Independent Variables — Physician Factors

Finally, several characteristics of the physician's background, practice setting, and hospital practice are specified in the models. Descriptive statistics for these measures are presented in table 2 for the three types of conditions studied here (medical, surgical, and maternity).

Table 2. Severity, patient, hospital and physician characteristics — univariate statistics by type of condition

	Medical Conditions		Surgical Conditions		Maternity Conditions	
	Mean	St. Dev	Mean	St. Dev	Mean	St. Dev
Physician Factors						
Years Experience	16.64	9.84	18.89	9.22	16.57	11.45
Internist (1=yes)	.86	.34	.06	.25	na	na
Surgeon (1=yes)	.01	.10	.93	.25	na	na
GP/FP (1=yes)	.10	.29	.00	.00	.13	.34
Board Certified (1=yes)	.75	.43	.85	.36	.71	.45
FMG (1=yes)	.22	.42	.09	.29	.10	.31
% Managed Care Practice	.16	.15	na	na	.13	.17
Log Volume of Patients	2.25	.44	2.60	.74	4.19	1.04
Concentration of Practice	.81	.24	.75	.25	.89	.22

Among the background characteristics, we include a continuous measure of the physician's experience (measured as the number of years since graduation from medical school), three dummy variables denoting the physician's speciality (internal medicine, surgery, general/family practice), dummy variables denoting board-certification and graduation from a foreign medical school, and (for U.S. and Canadian physicians) a classification variable indicating the particular medical school attended. There is some discretion in selecting the particular speciality variables to include in which models. In prior research, we have found that surgeons sometimes attend to internal medicine patients, while internists may attend to patients who have surgery. We therefore employed the following strategy in using the speciality variables. For the medical diagnoses, we included surgeon and general/family practice; for the surgical diagnoses, we included internist and general/family practice; and for the maternity diagnoses, we included only general/family practice.

To measure practice setting, we aggregated each physician's hospital caseload for a particular diagnosis by the patient's insurance coverage. The number of patients covered by managed care plans was divided by the total number of patients treated to derive a measure of the percent of practice that is managed care. Given the lower propensity of hospitalization for managed care patients, this is a conservative estimate of the physician's involvement in managed care.

Similar methods were used to describe the characteristics of the physician's hospital practice. We first aggregated the physician's admissions for a particular diagnosis across all hospitals utilized in order to develop a measure of the physician's hospital volume. Next, we computed a herfindal index to measure the concentration of admissions across all hospitals utilized. This index is the sum of the squared proportions of the physician's total admissions at each hospital in the market.

SOURCES OF DATA

The data required to conduct these analyses are taken from several sources. *Patient discharge data* are reported by hospitals to the Arizona Department of Health Services, which collates and disseminates the data to researchers. The data set includes only non-federal general and childrens hospitals with fifty or more beds (N=48). All federal (e.g. Veterans Administration, Department of Defence, Public Health Service), non-general (e.g. psychiatric), and general hospitals with less than fifty beds are excluded. Their exclusion does not seriously bias our findings for several reasons. First, the excluded hospitals account for only sixteen percent of all admissions to Arizona hospitals during the study period. Second, the excluded hospitals are unlikely sites where large numbers of patients in the medical and surgical diagnoses might be treated.

The state discharge database includes information on each patient's date of birth, gender, dates of admission and discharge, total charges, source of admission (e.g., emergency room), status of discharge (e.g., discharged to nursing home), DRG, principal and secondary diagnoses and procedures, insurance coverage, attending physician, and hospital utilized. In the present study, patient discharges cover the hospital reporting period from January 1st, 1989 to December 31st, 1990.

Three limitations of these data deserve some comment. First, the data pool managed care (HMO) and Blue Cross patients into one insurance category. Due to the high market penetration of managed care firms in the state (30.5% share in Pima County by 1990), this category may mask a pronounced managed care effect. Second, the data do not allow us to control for differences in payment mechanisms used by insurers to reimburse hospitals. As Melnick and Mann (1989) and Lave and Frank (1990) point out, observed differences in hospital charges may partly reflect different incentives imposed by the various payment mechanisms each insurer utilizes. Third, the total charges measure provides only a rough proxy of hospital resource use. It is not an exact measure of hospital costs; nor does it capture probable differences in the cost-to-charge ratios across hospitals. To correct for this latter problem, we incorporate a classification variable in the regression models to denote the specific hospital utilized.

Hospital data on hospital ownership, teaching affiliation, and facilities are coded from the *Annual Guide* published by the American Hospital Association (AHA, 1990; 1991). *Physician data* are coded from information provided by the state medical association. Using the physician's license number, we merged clinical information contained in the state discharge database with biographical information on each physician. Data on the physician's hospital practice characteristics were aggregated from patient records in the discharge data.

EMPIRICAL RESULTS

Contribution of Physician Factors to the Model

As our first aim, we assessed the power of the set of physician characteristics to explain variations in adjusted hospital charges. Table 3 decomposes the explained variation for each of the ten conditions. The first three columns present the R-square for regression models containing only severity and patient factors (Column 1), severity/ patient factors and a hospital identifier (column 2), and severity/patient factors and both hospital and physician identifiers (column 3) as predictors. The fourth column reports the F-statistic and significance for the increment in the explained variation due to the addition of the physician identifier (i.e., column three versus column two). Following Neter, Wasserman, and Kutner (1985), the F-statistic used to test the significance of the increment in explained variation is computed by

$$F = [(SSE_R - SSE_F)/(df_R - df_F)]/MSE_F$$

where SSE_R and SSE_F are the error sums of squares from the reduced and full models, df_R and df_F are the associated degrees of freedom, and MSE_F is the mean square error of the full model.

The results in Table 3 indicate that the incremental variation explained by the physician identifier is statistically significant in nine of the ten conditions. This finding confirms those reported earlier by Horn *et al* (1984) and Feinglass *et al*

Table 3. Variable in adjusted charges explained by patient, hospital and physician characteristics and significance of incremental variation explained by the addition of physician characteristics

Medical Conditions	R-Square for ANCOVA models incorporating			F-Test of Incremental Variation Explained
	Patient Factors	Hospital Identifier	Physician Identifier	
Chronic Obstructive Pulmonary Disease	.123	.168	.256	F = 1.69c
Myocardial Infarction	.209	.255	.318	F = 1.76c
Congestive Heart Failure	.123	.181	na	
Atrial Fibrillation	.112	.164	.230	F = 4.63c
Surgical Conditions				
Coronary Artery Bypass	.308	.325	.383	F = 2.62c
Large Bowel Resection	.175	.239	.302	F = 1.54a
Major Joint Procedures	.115	.134	.213	F = 5.77c
Hip Fracture	.145	.195	.245	F = 1.13
Maternity Conditions				
Caesarean Section	.100	.113	.164	F = 3.63c
Vaginal Delivery	.101	.117	.156	F = 10.58c

a: p < .05   b: p < .01   c: p < .001

(1991). Moreover, the addition of the physician identifier typically explains more incremental variation than the hospital identifier. This result is based on a conservative test of the power of physician effects, given that the physician identifier was added last to the model.

There is thus strong support for Hypothesis 1. This suggests that variations in physician practice style do indeed account for a significant amount of variation in hospital utilization, and can be linked to higher vs. lower efficiency in utilizing hospital services. Prior research has been unable to systematically identify *what* physician practice styles contribute to this variability, however. In the following section, we test hypothesized relationships of specific physician factors on utilization.

Hypothesized Effects of Physician Factors

To test the physician effects, we replaced the physician identifier with seven physician measures: experience, generalist, board-certified, foreign medical graduate (FMG), percentage of HMO patients in practice, patient volume in hospitals, and concentration of hospital practice. A final physician measure, the particular medical school attended, is omitted for the present due to missing information for several physicians; it is included in a subsequent model (see below).

Table 4 presents the parameter estimates from the regression model for each of the ten conditions. There is mixed support for the hypotheses regarding the effect of physician background characteristics. Contrary to Hypothesis 2, there is no clear-cut tendency for more experienced physicians to utilize hospital services more efficiently. Experience exhibits the expected negative relationship for two conditions, but significant positive relationships for two others. There is more support for Hypothesis 3. In three of the six conditions for which general/family practitioners are sometimes observed as the attending physician, generalist background exerts a significant, negative effect on utilization. There is less support for the effects of board certification (Hypothesis 4) and foreign medical training (Hypothesis 5). Not only are significant effects observed in only a minority of the conditions, but these few effects are mixed in their direction.

As a whole, the background factors appear to be neither powerful nor consistent predictors of hospital utilization. All of these characteristics are relatively fixed, given their prior formation during the physician's socialization. We conducted a more direct test of the socialization hypothesis (Hypothesis 6) by including a medical school identifier in an additional regression model and assessing the incremental variation explained over the type of model estimated in Table 4, but with the same number of observations (results not presented). The regression results indicate that the addition of medical school contributes a significant amount of additional explained variation in all but two of the conditions - both medical diagnoses (large bowel resection and hip fracture). The effect is remarkable in two ways. First, many researchers consider the post-graduate residency to be the more formative experience in the physician's socialization for subsequent practice behaviour. Second, the average years of experience of the physicians studied here is between sixteen and nineteen. This suggests that socialization forces not captured by the training and speciality measures already specified in the model do influence subsequent practice style years after graduation.

Estimates for the effects of the practice setting and hospital practice characteristics in table 4 are slightly more consistent, but not always in the expected direction. In support of Hypothesis 7, there is some indication that a greater share of managed care (HMO) patients in the physician's hospital practice is associated with more efficient utilization. This result holds regardless of the insurance coverage of the patient. Thus, physicians with more managed care patients seem to treat other patients more efficiently.

Contrary to Hypotheses 8 and 9, however, physicians with large patient volumes and hospital practices concentrated in one facility tend to utilize more rather than fewer services. The former result suggests that while greater experience with (i.e., volume of) similar cases may be associated with lower patient mortality (Hannan *et al* 1989), it is also associated with greater inefficiency in utilization. Physicians with heavier caseloads in a given diagnosis may be less able to manage these cases efficiently due to increased information processing requirements. The latter result suggests that while physicians may concentrate their practice in one hospital to maximize their own convenience and efficiency (Wholey and Burns 1991), they may not spend any more effort than other physicians in managing their cases efficiently. Indeed, the results suggest that they are less efficient.

CONCLUSION

In support of the growing literature on practice style, our findings identify the physician as a major source of variation in health care utilization. Characteristics of the physician's background, practice setting, and hospital practice are associated with the degree of efficiency in utilizing hospital services. The background characteristics exert less consistent effects than the others. They are also less mutable than the others in the short-term. Nevertheless, the results suggest greater effort might be devoted in the future to altering the socialization experiences of physicians in training. Such changes include encouraging the training of more generalists and teaching cost-efficient styles of practice in medical school and residency training. Neither of these suggestions is new.

The effect of practice setting on efficient utilization is consistent with the literature comparing HMOs with fee-for-service (Luft 1980; Dowd *et al* 1986; Johnson *et al* 1989). It is also consistent with studies showing that organizational factors exert a strong influence over the outcomes of care, both quality and cost (cf. Scott and Flood, 1984; Kelly and Hellinger, 1986; Burns and Wholey, 1991; Keeler, Rubenstein, Kahn *et al*, 1992). Taken together, these findings suggest that developing new practice settings and arrangements can encourage styles of practice that are both more efficient and higher quality.

Table 4. Impact of physician factors on adjusted hospital charges (std error in parentheses)

Medical Conditions	Experience	Gen/Family Practitioner	Board Certified	Foreign Med Grad	% HMO Practice
Chronic Obstructive Pulmonary Disease	-12.66 (13.28)	644.17 (591.07)	113.37 (267.48)	195.21 (272.65)	-305.70a (144.25)
Myocardial Infarction	3.49 (11.15)	-1236.13a (570.94)	-208.55 (240.87)	97.83 (199.36)	-0.36 (102.73)
Congestive Heart Failure	2.39 (5.80)	-654.05c (190.15)	149.54 (119.73)	364.87b (120.66)	-110.13 (65.48)
Atrial Fibrillation	-20.02a (10.01)	n/a	-641.47a (258.87)	324.62a (168.26)	-95.17 (87.51)
Surgical Conditions					
Coronary Artery Bypass	46.43 (58.87)	n/a	-4275 (3062)	2693a (1400)	554.93 (411.73)
Large Bowel Resection	-21.10 (30.60)	n/a	-150.97 (999.33)	2097.65b (790.58)	180.40 (307.75
Major Joint Procedures	00.95 (06.82)	3108.35 (2014.31)	-550.56b (188.62)	-435.15 (236.01)	-41.45 (64.23)
Hip Fracture	55.68a (23.70)	n/a	-826.30 (607.21)	844.49 (879.96)	116.83 (267.04)
Maternity Conditions					
Caesarean Section	-4.48c (1.06)	205.45 (114.4)	-9.47 (23.81)	-28.23 (27.95)	-80.90c (12.03)
Vaginal Delivery	0.72a (0.31)	-128.15c (20.10)	36.12c (7.44)	-67.52c 36.87c	-36.87c (03.87)

a: $p < .05$ b: $p < .01$ c: $p < .00$

n/a: General/family practitioners are not observed as the attending physician for these conditions, hence, there is no effect.

Medical Conditions	Physician Hosp Volume	Practice Concentration
Chronic Obstructive Pulmonary Disease	259.16 (167.59)	-895.31 (628.55)
Myocardial Infarction	249.67a (126.69)	318.03 (444.54)
Congestive Heart Failure	30.56 (79.34)	256.56 (270.46)
Atrial Fibrillation	-29.12 (135.10)	76.65 (372.09)
Surgical Conditions		
Coronary Artery Bypass	819.79a (423.64)	-206.33 (2221.52)
Large Bowel Resection	276.98 (380.50)	-2642.84a (12327.57)
Major Joint Procedures	556.82c (055.42)	929.89b (295.09)
Hip Fracture	815.48a (403.91)	1947.40 (1180.18)
Maternity Conditions		
Caesarean Section	20.90 (13.79)	297.53c (44.29)
Vaginal Delivery	-17.87c (03.75)	128.63c (13.67)

a: $p < .05$ b: $p < .01$ c: $p < .001$

The effect of the hospital practice characteristics is more troubling. If physicians are indeed motivated by income and convenience, as researchers have argued (cf. Pauly and Redisch, 1973; Feldstein, 1988; Wholey and Burns, 1991), then they should seek to increase their patient volume and concentrate their practice in one hospital. Both factors are found here to be associated with less efficient utilization. It is not clear what accounts for these effects, although we have proposed some possible explanations. Regardless, it will be difficult to mitigate these effects due to physicians' claims of professional autonomy and independence.

Our findings also have two important methodological implications for investigations of clinical practice variations. First, they suggest that practice style can be operationalized and modelled using available databases and measures to yield fairly consistent results. In particular, the characteristics of the physician's hospital practice are easily studied using databases that include physician identifiers. This type of research will help to uncover some of the reasons why physician identifiers exhibit a strong ability to explain variation in utilization.

Second, they suggest that socialization experiences, whether in medical school or residency programs, have important long-term influences that need to be investigated. Further study of the characteristics of the medical schools where physicians are trained (and the hospitals where residency programs are offered) is warranted.

REFERENCES

American Hospital Association. (1990), *Annual Guide*. Chicago: American Hospital Association.

American Hospital Association (1991), *Annual Guide*. Chicago: American Hospital Association.

Bosk, C. (1979), *Forgive and Remember*. Chicago: University of Chicago Press.

Burns, L.R., and Wholey, D.R. (1991), 'The Effects of Patient, Hospital, and Physician Characteristics on Length of Stay and Mortality', *Medical Care*, 29 (3), 251-271.

Burns, L.R., Wholey, D.R., and Huonker, J. (1991), 'Physician Use of Hospitals: Effects of Physician, Patient, and Hospital Characteristics'. *Health Services Management Research*, 2 (), 191-203.

Burns, L.R., Wholey, D.R., and Abeln, M. (1992), 'Using Managed Care to Mainstream the Poor: Hospital Utilization and Mortality Levels for Patients in the Arizona Health Care Cost Containment System'. Provisionally Accepted for Publication, *Inquiry*.

Childs, A.W., and Hunter, D. (1972), 'Non-Medical Factors Influencing Use of Diagnostic X-Ray by Physicians'. *Medical Care*, 10 (4), 323-335.

Chilingerian, J.A. (1989), 'Investigating Non-Medical Factors Associated with the Technical Efficiency of Physicians in the Provision of Hospital Services: A Pilot Study'. Paper Presented at Annual Meeting of Academy of Management, Washington D.C.

Chilingerian, J.A., and Glavin, M.P. (1992), 'Temporary Firms in Hospitals: Elements of a Managerial Theory of Clinical Efficiency'. Paper presented at Annual Meeting of Academy of Management, Las Vegas.

Coughlin, D., and Patel, V. (1987), 'Processing of Critical Information by Physicians and Medical Students'. *Journal of Medical Education*, 62 (), 818-829.

Cromwell, J., Mitchell, J.B., Calore, K.A., and Iezzoni, L. (1987), 'Sources of Hospital Cost Variation by Urban-Rural Location'. *Medical Care*, 25 (9), 801-829.

Dowd, B.E., Johnson, A.N., and Madson, R.A. (1986), 'Inpatient Length of Stay in Twin Cities Health Plans'. *Medical Care*, 24 (8), 694-710.

Eisenberg, J., and Nicklin, D. (1981), 'Use of Diagnostic Services by Physicians in Community Practice'. *Medical Care*, 19 (3), 297-309.

Eisenberg, J. (1986), *Doctors' Decisions and the Cost of Medical Care*. Ann Arbor, MI: Health Administration Press.

Feinglass, J., Martin, G.J., and Sen, A. (1991), 'The Financial Effect of Physician Practice Style on Hospital Resource Use'. *Health Services Research*, 26 (2), 183-205.

Feldstein, P.J. (1988), *Health Care Economics*. New York: John Wiley & Sons.

Fishbane, M., and Starfield, B. (1981), 'Child Health Care in the United States'. *New England Journal of Medicine*, 305 (), 552-556.

Flood, A.B., Scott, W.R., and Ewy, E. (1984), 'Does Practice Make Perfect? Part I: The Relation Between Hospital Volume and Outcomes for Selected Diagnostic Categories'. *Medical Care*, 22 (2), 98-114.

Fox, R.C. (1988), *Essays in Medical Sociology*. New Brunswick, NJ: Transaction Books.

Freeland, M.S., and Schendler, C.E. (1983), 'National Health Expenditure Growth in the 1980s: An ageing Population, New Technologies, and Increasing Competition'. *Health Care Financing Review*, 4 (3), 1

Galbraith, J. (1977), *Organization Design*. Reading, MA: Addison Wesley.

Goldfarb, M.G., Hornbrook, M.C., and Higgins, C.S. (1983), 'Determinants of Hospital Use: A Cross-Diagnostic Study'. *Medical Care*, 21 (1), 48-66.

Hannan, E.L., O'Donnell, J.F., Kilburn, H., et al. (1989), 'Investigation of the Relationship Between Volume and Mortality for Surgical Procedures Performed in New York State Hospitals'. *Journal of American Medical Association*, 262 (), 503.

Horn, S.D., and Sharkey, P.D. (1983), 'Measuring Severity of Illness to Predict Patient Resource Use Within DRGs'. *Inquiry*, 20 (4), 314-321.

Horn, S.A., Horn, R.A., and Sharkey, P.D. (1984), 'The Severity of Illness Index as a Severity Adjustment to Diagnosis-Related Groups'. *Health Care Financing Review*, Annual Supplement, 33-45.

Horn, S.D., Bulkley, G., Sharkey, P.D., Chambers, A.F., Horn, R.A., and Schramm, C.J. (1985), 'Interhospital Differences in Severity of Illness: Problems for Prospective Payment Based on Diagnosis-Related Groups (DRGs)'. *New England Journal of Medicine*, 313 (1), 20-24.

Hornbrook, M.C., and Goldfarb, M.G. (1981), 'Patterns of Obstetrical Care in Hospitals'. *Medical Care*, 19 (1), 55-67.

Jencks, S.K., and Kay, T. (1987), 'Do Frail, Disabled, Poor and Very Old Medicare Beneficiaries have Higher Hospital Charges?'. *Journal of the American Medical Association*, 257 (2), 198-202.

Johnson, A.N., Dowd, B., Morris, N.E., and Lurie, N. (1989), 'Differences in Inpatient Resource Use by Type of Health Plan'. *Inquiry*, 26 (3), 388-398.

Keeler, E.B., Rubenstein, L.V., Kahn, K.L., Draper, D., Harrison, E.R., McGinty, M.J., Rogers, W.H., and Brook, R.H. (1992), 'Hospital Characteristics and Quality of Care'. *Journal of American Medical Association*, 268 (13), 1709-1714.

Kelly, J.V., and Hellinger, F.J. (1986), 'Physician and Hospital Factors Associated with Mortality of Surgical Patients'. *Medical Care*, 24 (9), 785-800.

Lave, J.R., and Frank, R.G. (1990), 'Effect of the Structure of Hospital Payment on Length of Stay'. *Health Services Research* 25 (2), 327-347.

Luft, H.S. (1978), 'How do Health Maintenance Organizations Achieve Their Savings?'. *New England Journal of Medicine*, 298, 1336-1343.

Luft, H.S. (1980), 'Assessing the Evidence on HMO Performance'. *Milbank Memorial Fund Quarterly*, 58 (4).

Manu, P., and Schwartz, S.E. (1983), 'Patterns of Diagnostic Testing in the Academic Setting: The Influence of Medical Attendings' Subspecialty Training'. *Social Science and Medicine*, 17 (), 1339-1342.

McMahon, L.F., and Newbold, R. (1986), 'Variation in Resource Use Within Diagnostic-related Groups: The Effect of Severity of Illness and Physician Practice'. *Medical Care*, 24 (5), 388-397.

MEDSTAT. (1992), *The MEDSTAT Report*. Number 1.

Melnick, G.A., and Mann, J.M. (1989), 'Are Medicaid Patients More Expensive? A Review and Analysis', *Medical Care Review*, 46 (3), 229-253.

Neter, J., Wasserman, W., and Kutner, M.H. (1985), *Applied Linear Statistical Models*. Second Edition. Homewood, IL: Irwin.

Newhouse, J.P., Schwartz, W.B., Williams, A.P., and Witsberger, C. (1985), 'Are Fee-for-Service Costs Increasing Faster than HMO Costs?' *Medical Care*, 29 (7).

Pauly, M.V., and Redisch, M. (1973), 'The Not-for-Profit Hospital as a Physician's Co-operative'. *American Economic Review*, 63 (1), 87-99.

Roos, N.P., Flowerdew, G., Wajda, A., and Tate, R.B. (1986), 'Variations in Physicians' Hospitalization Practices: A Population-based Study in Manitoba, Canada'. *American Journal of Public Health*, 76 (1), 45-51.

Scott, W.R., and Flood, A.B. (1984), 'Costs and Quality of Hospital Care: A Review of the Literature'. *Medical Care Review*, 41 (Winter), 213-261.

Shortell, S.M., and LoGerfor, J.P. (1981), 'Hospital Medical Staff Organization and Quality of Care: Results for Myocardial Infarction and Appendectomy'. *Medical Care*, 19 (10), 1041-1053.

Thomas, J.W., and Ashcraft, M.L.F. (1991), 'Measuring Severity of Illness: Six Severity Systems and Their Ability to Explain Cost Variations'. *Inquiry* 28 (1), 39-55.

Wennberg, J.E., and Gittelsohn, A. (1975), 'Health Care Delivery in Maine: I. Patterns of Use of Common Surgical Procedures'. *Journal of Maine Medical Association*, 66, 123-130.

Wennberg, J.E., Barnes, B.A., and Zubkoff, M. (1982), 'Professional Uncertainty and the Problem of Supplier-Induced Demand'. *Social Science and Medicine*, 16, 811-824.

Wholey, D.R., and Burns, L.R. (1991), 'Convenience versus Independence: Do Physicians Strike a Balance in Their Admitting Decisions?' *Journal of Health and Social Behaviour*, 32, 254-272.

20 Changing Incentives in the Hospital Firm — An Experiment at Akershus Central Hospital, Norway

SVEIN PETTER RAKNES

Ministry of Health and Social Affairs, Norway

INTRODUCTION

Hospitals in Norway are mostly owned and funded by County Councils. The primary structure of the budgeting policy is built on 'frame budgeting'. This implies that each hospital is, along with an annual budgeting process, given an economic 'frame' related to production of often crudely specified bundles of services.

Akershus Central Hospital is owned by Akershus County. It treats approximately 22,000 in-patients and 80,000 out-patients per year. The 1992 budget was NOK 523 million (£ 45 million). In 1987 an experiment was set up to change the incentives and decentralize the management structure of the hospital. The major areas targeted for development in the project were:

1. To establish an explicit goal structure,
2. To define quality indicators,
3. To refine quantity measures,
4. To set up and evaluate an internal transfer pricing policy between hospital departments,
5. To establish hospital departments as 'profit centres',
6. To decentralize the operational decisions on a combination of input factors in the production, including staff management,
7. To introduce a new financing system based on reimbursement per patient treated. This was based on a decreasing willingness to pay for production which exceeded the production plans allocations.

The project ideas were developed in 1987-88. The actual experiment was carried out in 1989-90 and evaluated in 1991. This is the first paper to be presented abroad since the projects evaluatory report was completed.

Strategic Issues in Health Care Management. Edited by M. Malek, J. Rasquinha and P. Vacani
© 1993 John Wiley & Sons Ltd

This paper begins with the project's process and organization. This is then followed by a description of objectives 1 - 8 stated above. Those fields that have had the most impact on changing incentives, and decentralizing management are then explained. Finally, the lessons to be learned from the process dimension, and, the actual results obtained, are summed up.

PROJECT ORGANIZATION

The project was initiated by the hospital's management and represented by the general manager. A project manager was employed to further develop the hospital management's initiative. A steering committee of 10 members was established. Five of these constituted the hospital management, and five the labour unions. The general manager chaired the committee.

Initially, thirteen areas of development were proposed and discussed. As previously mentioned, a final eight areas were agreed upon. The strategic plan of the project encompassed these eight areas of development, and included timetables for activity to push these objectives.

The hospital staff were invited to take part in development teams. Around a hundred of them indicated interest, and were spread out evenly among the eight development areas. Through a 'delphi' process forty of these were allocated to eight development teams, five in each team. The 'delphi' process involved three independent senior members of the hospital staff (a chief consultant, head of the nurses unit for postgraduate training, and the head of the office for organizational development). These three members were given information on the candidates, the major challenges in each of the eight areas, and the timetable for each area. None of the three knew others identity. After two rounds of proposals, the team were close to consensus on the staffing of the eight development teams. This was sent to the steering committee which made marginal changes only. The final project plan which evolved from the eight development groups, was thereafter co-ordinated by the project manager and steering committee. The main part of this work was undertaken in 1988. Figure 1 indicates the structure of the project organization.

In 1989, the proposals accepted by the steering committee were applied, with the committee continually evaluating the process. Further, as an important part of the project process, external specialists were also employed to evaluate two dimensions of the project:

- Did the project effect the quality of the services provided by the hospital and the quality of the working conditions for the staff?
- Did the project effect the productivity of the hospital, ie. the volume of production compared to costs?

Two research institutes, both closely related to health services research, were chosen from a number of research and consultancy firms that were assessed.

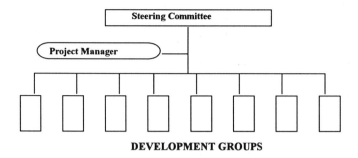

Figure 1. The project organisation

THE OBJECTIVES IN VIEW

Defining an explicit goal structure

The objective of the project was to improve the hospital's health service provision for a given resource input. The principal goal structure developed for the hospital had two dimensions.

1. The functional areas covered:

- Service related goals
- Administrative, organizational and staff oriented goals

2. The time perspective examined:

- Long term goals and visions;
- Annual strategic goals (often called strategic plans) to achieve the long term goals and visions, and;
- Lists of actions with specifications e.g. person in charge and time tables specified on dates and weeks.

This objective attempted to identify a set of long term goals as a basis for the annual strategic planning process. The normative basis of the goal-document was to combine services of excellence in a strong atmosphere of dignity. The areas covered were:

- Accessibility
- High quality diagnostic work in close co-operation with the patient
- Equal treatment for equal cases based on a positive capacity to benefit
- Treatment and care is given to maximise quality of life as well as post treatment life expectancy

- Managerial development including goal setting on departmental level.

An evaluation of how well the goal structure had been communicated to hospital staff, and whether it had effected the production was carried out. The results indicated an increased awareness of, and commitment to, the goal of the programme during the project period. However, the problems involved in measuring this area were significant, and thus, one is unable to draw any strong conclusions.

Quality indicators

Quality measurement was concentrated in two regions:

- The technical quality of the services
- The human relations quality of the services.

Three characteristics were required for the quality indicator:

- Relevance
- Quantifiability
- Simplicity (easy to collect and understand)

Quality indicators were developed for the following five areas:

- Admitting patients to the hospital
- Diagnostic work
- Medical treatment
- Care
- Discharging patients from the hospital

Thirteen indicators were developed and implemented. One of the most interesting areas developed was optical readable patient questionnaires. The systematic interviewing of the consumers of services is important. This is particularly the case when there is no market mechanism to respond to quality improvements, both because of the restricted freedom of choice, and, because of the strong tradition of provider defined quality (based on the asymmetric information argument).

Most of the quality indicators were deemed positive, i.e. as efficient means of measurement. They were:

1. *Admission*
   - Capacity to deal with emergency cases, beds at disposal.
   - The admission date compared with the pre admission priority setting for each patient. (emergency, within 24 hours, one week, one month and "waiting list").

2. *Diagnosis*
   - Reports from post-mortem investigations.
3. *Treatment*
   - Cases reported to the committee investigating hospital injuries
   - Quality tests on patient files
   - The updating of knowledge
4. *Care*
   - Waiting time from the patient is admitted to the first action in terms of diagnostic work or treatment
   - Patient information
   - The patients' contact with the outside world and with the hospital staff
   - The food
   - A patient survey
5. *Leaving the hospital*
   - Timing discharge
   - Documentation of the patient and GP at the point of discharge.

Quantity indicators

These indicators were developed from the original hospital statistics based on the ICD-9 classification. For each major speciality a report based on diagnostic groups was developed. This indicated 15-20 groups per speciality, reporting on the number of patients discharged, the number of bed days, the average length of stay, the number of emergency cases, and the surgical activity. This process was a step towards implementing Diagnostic Related Groups (DRGs) to measure changes in case-mix (an indicator of changes in workload per patient treated). The project thus introduced DRGs, which were used in the evaluation of its outcome.

Combining case-mix with the number of patients treated, allow a better understanding of the hospital as a multi product firm. It also provides a more precise empirical basis for the pricing and budgeting process when compared to traditional measures. This is positive for both, the intra hospital process, (e.g. the departmental budgets and production planning), and, for the external process (negotiating production volume and budgets with the county council).

Transfer pricing

The reasons for implementing transfer pricing policies were because it was argued that it was more efficient to obtain optimal production and allocation of intermediate goods and services if the 'demand side' was confronted with the cost of the product. This was in contrast to a centralized allocation policy regulated through the annual budgeting process. The key question was which system had the lowest transaction costs. The implementation of new information technology (IT) has made a major contribution to the reduction of transaction costs related to establishing 'internal markets' within the hospital firm. In meetings with hospital staff, two lines of problems were examined:

- In order to be able to give the departments supplying intermediate products status as "decision centres" or 'profit centres', transfer pricing would be a necessary condition.
- For the clinical decision maker the value of the opportunity forgone by demanding an extra set of tests, without knowing and paying the production cost is unclear,and probably in most cases perceived as nil..

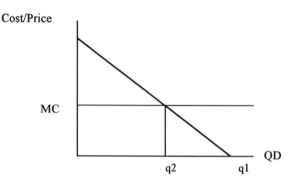

Figure 2. Excess demand for a zero priced good

If the price faced is zero, one can expect the quantity demanded to be q^1. If the price reflects the marginal cost of producing an extra unit, the quantity demannded would be expected to be q^2. An important assumption here is that the representative for the demand side is informed about prices and her/his department is responsible for its own budget, and acts accordingly.

The experiment was applied for microbiology. The pricing policy involved:[1]

- An agreement between the supply side and the demand side (the clinical departments) on the expected level of demand for the year to come.
- Average cost pricing according to this agreement, and,
- Any deviation from the agreement was priced on a marginal cost basis.

The evaluation showed that all departments apart from gynaecology/obstetrics had a decreasing demand for the services involved. The reductions were not large, but they changed the previous years trend towards increasing demand.

---

[1] A firm list of pricing policies was discussed in the hospital (referred in a paper presented for the U.K. HESG in July 1988, Raknes 1988), and based in Hirsleifer (1956), Brown & Jaques (1964) and Bruzelius (1987). This is more extensively discussed in Raknes (1989); available on request from the author.

Departments as decision/profit centres

Decentralizing management decisions within a firm is frequently discussed in the management literature. When a firm grows, it will at some point be faced with problems of sub-optimization and sub-cultures. These can either be viewed as a control and steering problem for the central office, or, one can develop, an incentive structure inviting departments to match their local goals with the firm's overall objective function. In examining hospitals as a firm there is a tradition for centralized control- mechanisms in the administrative part of the firm, and decentralized management for clinical decisions (clinical freedom) in the medical section of the firm. Thus, the objective is not only to decentralize, but also to obtain a more conformed strategy in clinical decisions. This was achieved by combining the clinical decision making and the economics of health care production. The medical and administrative parts of the hospital firm (Harris, 1977) were merged to become one firm with departments as the most important basis for decision making through the year[2]. However, once annually, the total strategy for the hospital was discussed and decided upon (a process covering several weeks). Within the frame of this 'corporate strategy' the departments could develop their own goals, negotiate production plans, and budget with the central office. Each department signed an agreement with the general manager, the long term perspective of which was to involve the clinical departments in the process with the central office. The service departments, however, serve the clinical departments, and should negotiate deals directly with the 'demand side' and not with the central office. We developed a 'profit sharing policy' as displayed in table 1.

Table 1. Profit sharing between departments and the central office.[3]

Result	Hospital Profit	Hospital Deficit
Department profit - department keeps	50%	25%
Department Deficit - department covers	50%	100%

The profit sharing model was developed to be as simple as possible, and to include an incentive to gain profit without transferring costs over to other departments. The problem with the model is the incentive to break-even rather than profit, because half the profit would be shared with the unit general manager, and thus not necessarily ploughed back into the department where it was generated.

---

2 The main strategy at the hospital was to make each department a team which was responsible for its own results both regarding production (quantity and quality) and economy. The central management and the departmental managers made a formalized agreement including production level and the budget plan. The agreement was signed by the departmental managers and the general manager.

3 To keep its profit, a department must fulfil its production plan. The rules were not perfectly symmetric, but they gave the central management a sum of money as a means of "strategic power".

Conversely, generating profit allows extra degrees of freedom in spending the money. Thus, departments could, for example, plan investments with the local staff

From mid 1988 to the end of 1989 the economic result changed from a loss of NOK 20 million to a profit of approximately NOK 19 million In 1990, the departments had at their disposal NOK 9.4 million, apart from the ordinary budget. Very few departments showed a loss.

However, as commented upon earlier, the tax income in the county has been lowered, which has in turn imparted severe constraints on hospital budgets. As a consequence of this 'depression', there has also been difficulties in the profit sharing model within the hospital.

Decentralized management of input factor mix

In the Norwegian public sector there is a tradition of a clear distinction between capital inputs and labour inputs in production. It has been difficult within the budget year, to switch money between these fields, and indeed, managers have had little freedom in changing staffing plans. The project in carrying out this objective proposed that:

i.   the County Council should:

   •   on behalf of the population define the spectrum and volume of services demanded.
   •   ensure efficient provision of the quality of services.

ii.   and the hospital's mission is to:

   •   provide high quality services within the framework agreed with the County Council. How this work is undertaken (i.e. how input factors are mixed) is a hospital management task, not a political issue.

The concrete areas under view related to staff management. The project proposal attributed to the hospital management full responsibility for the staff management, the number of staff hired, changes in the mix of professionals, and if deemed necessary, reductions of staff.

This was instinctively challenged by the trade unions, and after negotiations between County Council representatives and the unions, a compromise result was reached. A hospital internal board consisting of the central management (five) and representatives for the trade unions (four) was given the responsibility for these decisions.

This board commenced work in 1989. The evaluation of its progress after two years was negative, and in the evaluation report it was recognized that one should either: return to the old decision structure, which entrusted the political Board for Somatic Hospitals in the county of Akershus the decision power; or, take the next step and give the General Manager the decisive and executive power to deal with the situation.

A new financing system

The objective of the project at this point was to:

- focus on the need for a more clearly developed purchaser - provider split.
- improve the incentive structure on the provider side.

The hospital (provider) should negotiate with the County Council (purchaser) to obtain an agreement covering the range of services the hospital was expected to provide, and at what cost to the purchaser. The County Council would represent the publics interest to negotiate the best buy of services, in view of the expressed medical need and the (monetary) purchasing power available. Instead of an annual budget proposal to the politicians, negotiations were undertaken between the hospital management and politicians around the same table. The negotiations attempted to reach a written agreement on the number of cases treated, the case mix (in-patient and out-patient), and the price for the purchaser providing these services.

The financing model had a prospective fixed price per case within the frame of the agreement. If the hospital provided more services than planned, the purchaser's willingness to pay decreased (figure 3).

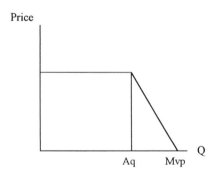

Q: Quantity   Aq: Agreed quantity   Mvp: Maximum willingness to pay

Figure 3. The financing model for inpatient services

If the quantity produced increases over and above Aq, the price paid per extra case by the purchaser decreased rapidly. If the production was less than agreed, the provider would experience reduced income. The excess prices are shown in table 2[4]:

---

4 The proposal was 2 percent intervals, i.e. giving a price > 0 for services up to 1,06 of the agreement.

Table 2. Excess prices

Deviation from agreememt	Price in percent of agreed price
1% (ie. up to 101%)	0.75
2% (ie. 101-102%)	0.5
3% (ie. 102-103%)	0.25
103% of plan and above	0

For outpatient services there was a fixed price per case independent of number of cases. In the first year of the experiment the results were as displayed in table 3:

Table 3. Excess prices

Services	Plan	Result
In-patients	21,650	22,472
Out-patients	69,000	78,112

This totalled a NOK 7.5 million value of 'extra' production according to the terms of the agreement. However, when this result reached the political system, financial crisis emerged to darken in the sky. The consequence was the extra money owed was never paid by the purchasing authority, bringing the project into some state of discredit.

Internal marketing

The mission of the internal marketing process was to inform as many of the hospital staff as possible about the ideas and contents of the project. It also attempted to involve those needed to advocate the project, and educate those in need of further competence, to execute high quality management in the new setting. The activities included:

- Monthly newsletters;
- Articles published in the hospitals internal newspaper;
- Seminars;

     i. General information seminars,
     ii. IT, basic course,
     iii. he application of DRGs,
     iv. The new budgeting system for departments,

- Information given in staff meetings in all departments;
- Information given in the monthly meetings for the departmental managers;
- Bringing the theme on the agenda in the annual management conferences (reaching approximately 150 personnel in management positions);
- Distributing all written material proposed for the steering group to the local representatives of the labour unions;
- Printing and distributing folders and posters covering the main philosophy of the project.

The evaluation concluded that even though the list of internal marketing activities was long, the project would have improved its performance if a large part of the staff had been better informed. Indeed, the success of organizational change depends heavily on well informed participants.

LESSONS TO BE LEARNED

The process

To continue from the previous comments in the objectives, internal marketing is essential favourably information and education of the staff, particularly in inspiring people to dedicate themselves to the changes being implemented rather than fighting them.

The structure of the project which involved a wide range of the hospital staff, was a success. Attempts to open a back door and, throw difficult issues over to the County Council was not as successful. However, this was part of the framework facing the project, independent of the local view in the hospital concerned.

The steering committee performed well in most cases when making necessary decisions. One question *ex post* is whether the consistency between the ideology of the project and the ideology of the day to day management was compatible, and well spelled out. This is the classical challenge regarding the interface between project management process involved in developing new paths for decision making, and new incentives, and, the day to day decision making process, even when the people involved are the same actors.

The development teams responded well, and produced excellent reports which included good background analysis and skilful recommendations for implementation. The National Institute of Public Health concluded that the project process had improved motivation among staff. They also observed an increased knowledge and awareness of the hospital goals, the results obtained, and the cost of production.

The results

The objective of the project was to maximise the hospital outcome for a given resource input. In evaluating if this was obtained, we attempted to analyse change in resource input, changes in output, and, changes along the quality-dimension.

The input-output analysis was performed by the Norwegian Institute of Hospital Research. A DRG-based model was applied to handle the case-mix changes. The case-mix adjusted volume of production (also controlled for re-admittance rates) increased by approximately 1 percent from 1988 to 1989, and by 3 percent from 1989 to 1990. The volume of out-patient services also increased, but for this part of the production we have no case-mix adjusting analysis.

In 1988 the overall cost index for the hospital was 10.7% above the national average. In 1989 it had fallen to 4.3%, and in 1990 it was 6.6% Controlled for the delay of some investments form 1988 to 1990, the change in index can be interpreted as being approximately 5% over the two years.

The National Institute of Public Health did not find any indications of reduced quality of the services provided by the hospital. In terms of quality in a wider perspective however, some improvements were introduced, routine patient surveys being one example.

The productivity of the hospital, however, was improved (evaluation carried out by the Hospital Research Institute, Trondheim). The DRG cost index was reduced from 1.107 in 1988 to 1.043 in 1990.

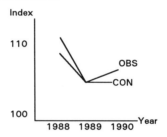

OBS: Observed changes
CON: Tendency when the changes were controlled for the delay of investments from 1988 to 1990.

Figure 4. Changes in cost index.

The main problem during the last project year was the reduction of the county's willingness to pay as a consequence of decreasing tax income. This led to a breakdown in the new financing system, and, a significant problem with de-motivation among the health care professionals in the hospital.

CONCLUSION

The project involved a wide range of the hospital staff in development teams. This process had an positive impact in the hospital. The changes initiated through the project also received a positive response in the evaluation, though there were shortfalls such as the establishment of an internal board for staff management decisions.

As a part of the management development strategy, the project was a positive exercise. Indeed, the ability to perform experiments and deal with changes is itself an important organizational quality.

REFERENCES

Beske, F. et al. (1987), *Hospital Financing Systems. Report on two WHO workshops.* Institute fur Gesundheits-System-Forschung, Kiel.

Brown, W. and Jaques, E. (1964), *Product Analysis Pricing.* Hainemann, London .

Bruzelius, N. (1987), *Om internpriser på medisinska servicetjenester.* Presented at the Nordic HESG-meeting, Åbo, 1987.

Harris J.E. (1977), *The Internal Organization of Hospitals: Some Economic Implications.* Bell Journal of Economics, 467-82.

Hirshleifer, J. (1956), *On the economics of Transfer Pricing.* Journal of Business, 172-84.

Raknes, S.P. (1988), *Management by objectives and Clinical Budgeting.* Presented at the HESG-meeting at Brunel University, July 1988.

Raknes, S.P. (1989), *How elements of Market Structure can be used to change Incentives in the Hospital Firm.* Presented at the Nordic HESG-meeting, Iceland, August 1989.

21 Managing Quality Assurance in German Hospitals — Approaches, Obstacles, Prospects

W. SATZINGER[1], K. PIWERNETZ[2] & J. JOHN[1]

[1]GSF-Institut für Medizinische Informatik und Systemforschung, Germany
[2]Gesundheitsreferat der Landeshauptstadt München, Germany

Quality assurance (QA) in medical care has quite a tradition. It can be traced back to those ancient health experts like Hippocrates who urged all persons working in the medical field to continuously assess what they are doing, and to ensure that, on balance, the benefits of their actions on, and for, the patients clearly outweigh the harm they might be causing to them.

Modern QA is, in its origin, primarily an American venture. After preparatory work in the field by proponents such as Codman (1914) and Lee and Jones (1933), it was conceptualised in the 1960s by Donabedian (from whom, among other things, we owe the basic distinction between quality of structure, of process and of outcome). The subject was then addressed by a number of other scholars: Williamson, Juran, Luft, Brook, to name but a few.

The fact that most of the of academic as well as practical work on QA has so far come from the U.S.A., is no mere accident. It was in the U.S.A. where the principle of systematic output control - a long-standing practice in industrial production - was first applied to the service sector in general and to health services in particular; and where, much earlier than elsewhere, the health care system came to be regarded as having an important economic dimension thus becoming subject to economical, rather than medical reasoning alone. There were two waves of development in this direction which helped to promote a quest for QA in health care (Wyszewianski 1988):

- First, starting in the sixties, when a tremendous expansion of services was followed by an enormous rise in health care expenditure;
- Second, in the late eighties, when severe cost containment measures led to a marked reduction of health services.

Strategic Issues in Health Care Management. Edited by M. Malek, J. Rasquinha and P. Vacani
© 1993 John Wiley & Sons Ltd

In both cases, the measurement of quality of care became crucial to finding the balance between resources and benefits: (1) Is the health care system worth the amount of money spent on it? (2) Is so little money sufficient to keep the system working in a satisfactory manner?

Obviously, in this context, the concept of 'quality' clearly exceeds what used to be its traditional meaning in medical care, namely the mere technical quality of certain services. It now also comprises, as essential elements, the medical appropriateness of such services as well as the human dimension of the ways in which they are delivered (Brook 1991).

Although in (West) Germany the situation has remained constant with regards to the development of health policy during the last decades (expansion of services and expenses, followed by efforts of cost containment), QA had played no significant role until the late 1980s. In contrast, in Great Britain and the Netherlands the American QA-debate had been addressed 15 to 20 years ago, and resulted in an impressive number of QA-projects and comprehensive QA-programmes, carried out by specially designed institutions. The West German health care system, on the other hand, and like the French one, has kept away from QA almost completely (Symposium 1991).

Notable exceptions, however, were: a study on perinatal care, set up locally in 1975 and mushrooming into a nationwide programme later on; attempted technical guidelines concerning the performance of laboratory tests, and preventive measures relating to the equipment required for some specialist services in ambulatory practices, the regular control of hygienic measures and of the handling of certain instruments in hospitals (Sachverständigenrat 1989). But all these were minor undertakings compared to the definition and need for QA in medical care.

Why is it then that, up until recently, QA has played such a marginal role in a country which justifiably prides itself on having one of the best health care and health insurance systems in the world? The main reason for this is that quality-related thinking in Germany is extremely structure-biased; this means that the cure for any deficiency observed is first and foremost sought for in the structure of the health care system (e.g. reform of medical schools in view of the great mass of students, reform of the nursing profession's image and profile with a view to attract more people to it), but much less in its working process. In principle, one can also say that most German health professionals are still so convinced of the excellence of their training and the high standard of their care institutions that they see no urgent need for special efforts to describe, analyze and evaluate in detail what is actually being performed. In other words, they still place so much trust in the quality of the structure of the care system that they fail to examine closely the quality of its process and outcome.

In German hospitals, for example, there exists a three-tier system of medical staff: young doctors, supervised by senior physicians who, in turn, are supervised by the medical head of department. For instance, contrary to the situation in many American hospitals, all these people are employees of the hospital, are permanently present there, and are supposed to be in constant contact with each other. As medicine is an experience-based practice rather than a full-blown science, so the argument goes, an optimal level of QA is already achieved, as long as the more experienced and competent members of staff are in a position to monitor and control the work of those less experienced, lower ranked ones. This system, allegedly, is guaranteed by the three-tier organization of medical staff. The same is, also true of the nursing staff; the addition being that nurses are also under the control of the physicians around them.

The assumption behind this arrangement is that such a system of competence and control within hospital staff is a guarantee for good performance, which means to say that the existence of a well-conceived structure must, more or less automatically, lead to a smooth working process and a high-quality outcome of hospital care.

Although this assumption seems to be sustained by the majority of the medical profession in Germany, in the last few years, a growing number of health politicians and specialists realized that considerably more would have to be done to prove the allegedly good quality of hospital services or even to improve it. Slowly but surely, QA in Germany became a health policy issue, and some action was taken in this respect.

- In 1986, the German Hospital Association and the Federal Chamber of Physicians agreed in principle to closely cooperate in the introduction of QA measures into hospital care.
- In 1988, the Chamber of Physicians declared that participation in QA was to be a professional duty for all German doctors.
- Most important, in 1989, the German Parliament passed a Health Reform Act which stated that all hospitals were obliged to take up QA-measures pertaining to the process of care as well as to the quality and effects of treatment. The Act also allows for comparisons between hospitals in this respect. The particulars of such programmes, says the law, are to be elaborated in contracts between hospital owners and health insurance funds.

These new developments in German health policy are certainly in part a reaction to events abroad, in countries like the U.S.A., Great Britain and the Netherlands; and the fact that, in distinguished journals and in international conferences, QA had become a major subject of discussion. In addition, the World Health Organization-Europe, in its programme Health For All 2000, published in 1984, had advanced QA by stating (target 31) that 'by 1990 all Member States should have built effective mechanisms for ensuring quality of patient care within their health care systems'.

The movement for paying increased attention to quality may also be seen as a reflection of the growing awareness that there exist unacceptable differences between individual health care institutions or even whole regions in terms of the level of quality of care or, at least, that there is a lack of standards against which the provision of health services can be measured and such differences could be assessed. Finally, and probably most decisive, it is an effect of the ever-growing pressure on care providers to demonstrate the effectiveness of their services and to increase their efficiency.

So, in any case, attempts have been made in recent years to put QA on the agenda of German health politics. And, indeed, several symposia were held and publications made on the subject, declarations of intent increased considerably in number and intensity. But in real terms not much has changed. A few new quality circles of physicians in ambulatory care have been established. Further; a handful of German Länder (the regional states) have amended their hospital laws with calls for QA; and, to be sure, a couple of pilot projects have been started - a short description of the two outstanding ones are necessary.

One pilot project on QA in hospitals was carried out in the northernmost state of Germany - Schleswig-Holstein (Niemann 1992). There, the regional Hospital Association and health insurance funds had entrusted a research institute with the task of organizing the development and testing of QA measures. Twelve out of about 130 hospitals, representing about 20 % of all hospital beds in the region, volunteered for participation in the project, which ran for a period of 18 months.

In order to design QA-studies, working groups of physicians were established, one for each of the following areas of hospital care: surgery, internal medicine, gynaecology/obstetrics and haemotherapy. In their meetings, these groups first picked out tracer diagnoses (like inguinal hernia) and general problems (such as nosocomial infections) to be tackled as specific subjects. They then developed common protocols (usually questionnaires) for the collection of relevant data. The organization of data collection was left to the individual hospitals. From them, the data was handed over to the institute to be processed. The resulting comparative statistics were finally fed back to the hospitals for further consideration.

Although the institute tried hard to motivate and instruct the staff concerned, to organize the implementation of the studies effectively, and to make extensive use of whatever could be established as a fact or finding, the end result of the whole undertaking does not seem very encouraging. Some topics of action turned out to be unsuitable or of high priority; much of the data gathered was not complete, reliable or valid enough to permit comparative assessments, and changes in the quality-relevant attitude and behaviour of staff, as far as they were intended and even achieved, hardly proved to be stable over time. It was a big effort for a small achievement.

This is not untypical of the sort of approach to QA that is called 'external QA'. With that, one will always have the problem that people experience QA either as a purely scientific exercise similar to therapy studies (but with no academic honours to gain) or as a wasteful action with a rather intransparent aim. It can also be viewed as a crude measure of insidious work control and, as an additional burden on their daily work. QA, they feel, is something certainly not in their interest to pursue.

The other major pilot project, worth mentioning, is the QA initiative by the City of Munich, owner of five hospitals, with 4,350 beds and about 6,800 members of staff. The project was called 'Trust through Quality', and it is described as a model of 'internal quality assurance with external support' (Piwernetz 1991).

Contrary to what is usually associated with QA in hospitals (expert commissions coming into the institution, collecting certain data on specific diagnostic or therapeutic procedures and comparing them to given standards, i.e. the "classical" retrospective chart audit approach to QA), the Munich strategy is about triggering a process of self-evaluation and self-regulation within the hospital, trying to involve all members of staff, irrespective of their profession or position.

Profiting from experience in the Netherlands over the last decade (witness the activities of CBO; see Reerink 1983), this strategy was developed by a small group of QA-experts working with the City's Health Department. Its main features are as follows:

As a principle, every one is responsible for the quality of his or her own work. By consequence, QA-activities have to start at the basic staff level. Physicians, nurses, lab assistants, administrative and technical staff members, are all required

- to document and analyze their daily work in order;
- to trace whatever appears to be a quality-relevant shortcoming;
- and then discuss such problems (and look for solutions) with their peers and, if necessary, with the higher ranks of hospital management.

It is primarily a process from starting from the bottom and working to the top; and for a start, everything is kept intra-mural (this is what is meant by internal QA). However, in the long run one cannot properly assess the quality of one's own work without referring to the quality standards of one's own profession; comparisons are needed with the peers in other hospitals. So, the process from the bottom to the top has to be complemented by a process from the inside to the outside, the internal transparency of the beginning will have to become external in the end.

In order to fulfil this task, it is clear, that hospital staff need a measure of external support; help in general orientation and a lot of assistance in methodological matters. This would enable them:

- to find the relevant information on criteria and indicators;
- to establish appropriate standards;
- to design sound QA projects or studies, and;
- to evaluate properly the effects of the QA-measures taken.

It is beyond the remit of this paper to describe, in any detail, the institutional and organizational arrangements that have been made to implement this strategy in Munich's five hospitals. However, for a rough idea, a typified process of the interactions necessary for the development and execution of a particular QA measure is depicted in figure 1 below.

- In the middle of it, the main actors are shown: the three QA-Agents (one each for the medical, nursing and administrative staff of each hospital) and the QA-Commission, consisting of the latter as well as of the three-headed hospital directorate and six delegates (physicians and nurses in equal numbers) from the three main sectors of the hospital (comprising the departments of surgery, of internal medicine and of biotechnical services);

- The first task of the QA-Agents is to stimulate, among their colleagues (right column), an awareness for quality problems and for the necessity of QA. This, hopefully, leads to staff discussions on the process and outcome of care activities. Any problems that emerge from there, are then to be reported - via the QA-Agents or the sector's representatives — to the QA-Commission.

- By the Commission, meeting about four times a year, those problems are to be brought into a priority order according to their importance/urgency and tractability. Then specific QA-project ideas are generated there and fed back to the respective sections of staff, where special project groups are to be established and to work on the problems in concern. The results of those projects will then be reported back to the Commission for concluding assessment.

- During the whole process, the hospital people receive considerable support from the Health Department's QA-Group (left column), which consists of medical, nursing and documentary specialists as well as a programme manager, headed by the programme director (who was also the leading figure in the development of the strategy). In combination with three internationally renowned QA-experts as temporary advisers, this group functions as a "backstopper" to the QA-actors and -activities in the hospitals, mainly by providing QA-relevant information, further education/training and some coordinating services.

This is the Munich concept of QA in hospitals admittedly in very broad terms. What should have become clear, nevertheless, is that, in its strategic approach this programme is similar to what is nowadays called 'total quality management' (Kaltenbach 1991). Thus, it is a far cry from the traditional design of 'external QA', which still dominates the approach to QA in German hospitals. It starts from the needs and observations of the very people who are working in that environment, motivates them to engage in comprehensive assessment of their own doing, stimulates them to find out what their standards could and should be, and urges them to look for steady improvement of the conditions, the processes and the results of their work.

Whether the Munich QA-model will succeed, remains, two years after its start, still to be seen. Its achievements so far are by no means negligible. The programme has managed to obtain and maintain the support of the City Council and of the local health insurance funds (which are financing it). It has also attracted some publicity that is well beyond municipal boundaries. In addition, quite a number of committed and well-trained personnel are geared to tackling quality problems in those five hospitals, and dozens of QA-measures diverse in scope and purpose, have already been carried out with respectable results.

On the other hand, the implementation of the programme has encountered, and is still faced with, a lot of difficulties. In part, they arise from the general crisis most German hospitals are presently in (shortage of resources, particularly of nursing

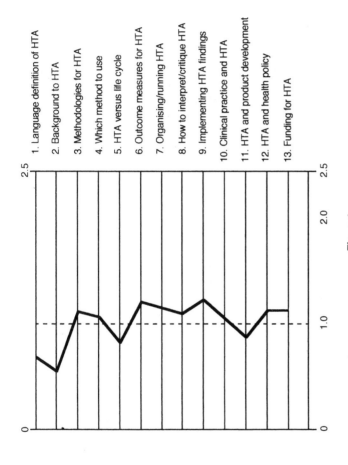

1. Language definition of HTA
2. Background to HTA
3. Methodologies for HTA
4. Which method to use
5. HTA versus life cycle
6. Outcome measures for HTA
7. Organising/running HTA
8. How to interpret/critique HTA
9. Implementing HTA findings
10. Clinical practice and HTA
11. HTA and product development
12. HTA and health policy
13. Funding for HTA

Figure 1

staff), which makes them rather reluctant to take on new tasks. An even more important obstacle, however, seems to be the hierarchic structure of hospital organization (especially the autocratic manner in which the higher ranks of personnel still deal with the lower ones, and many physicians with the nurses), which, of course, stands in sharp contrast to the participatory approach of this QA-strategy.

At the moment, the odds are not very much in favour of the Munich QA-model. It may have too little time to prove its potential for success and, therefore, might not survive politically. But if it fails, a good chance for sound quality assurance in inpatient care will be lost.

REFERENCES

Brook, R.H. (1991), 'Quality of Care: Do we Care?', *Annals of Internal Medicine*, 115 (6), 486-490.

Codman, E.A. (1914), 'The Product of a Hospital', *Surgery, Gynecology and Obstetrics*, 18 (1914), 491-496.

Kaltenbach, T. (1991), *Qualitätsmanagement im Krankenhaus*, Bibliomed, Melsungen.

Lee, R.I. and Jones, L.W. (1933), *The Fundamentals of Good Medical Care*, University of Chicago Press, Chicago.

Niemann, F. and Beske, F. (1992), *Qualitätssicherung in Krankenhäusern Schleswig-Holsteins*, Institut für Gesundheits-System-Forschung, Kiel.

Piwernetz, K., Selbmann, H.-K., Vermeij, D. (1991), '"Vertrauen durch Qualität". Das Münchner Modell der Qualitätssicherung im Krankenhaus', *Das Krankenhaus* 11, 558.

Reerink, E., *Quality assurance in the Netherlands*, CBO, Utrecht.

Sachverständigenrat für die Konzertierte Aktion im Gesundheitswesen (1989), *Qualität, Wirtschaftlichkeit und Perspektiven der Gesundheitsversorgung, Jahresgutachten 1989*, Nomos, Baden-Baden.

Symposium zur Qualitätssicherung (1991), *Teil 1: Stationäre und ambulante medizinische Versorgung*, Bundesminister für Arbeit und Sozialordnung (ed), Forschungsbericht Nr. 203, Bonn.

Wyszewianski, L. (1988), 'Quality of Care: Past Achievements and Future Challenges', *Inquiry* 25, 13-22.

22 A Contract Negotiation Simulation Experiential Learning Workshop for Clinical Directors and an Acute Hospital Management Board

JILL SCHOFIELD

Aston Business School

INTRODUCTION

Negotiation is not new to the National Health Service (NHS) in the UK. Indeed, it could be argued that the creation of the NHS was a result of compromises reached, from a series of negotiations, in a mixed motive environment between various political, ideological and professional groups (Willcocks 1967). Nor is the experience of some sort of trading agreement between health authorities new, albeit that these agreements were more often the result of bilateral negotiations which were not highly formalised. In their 1989 study of such trading in clinical services, the National Association of Health Authorities (NAHA) and Newcastle Polytechnic described the process of agreeing the basis for a contract, not as one derived from a "clean cut evaluation,....but much messier" (Appleby, Middlemas and Ranade 1989).

Managerial expertise in contract negotiation and service specification tended to be more developed in those professionals who traditionally dealt with external contractors, such as engineers, supplies officers and catering managers. The advent of competitive tendering in 1983 for a range of support services, especially in hospitals, introduced a formal element of contract negotiation into the health care environment. It also served to widen the net of expertise in negotiation skills to other groups of professionals and workers, including general managers. However, the publication of the White Paper, *Working For Patients* (1989), and the subsequent *NHS and Community Care Act* (1990), heralded the advent of a trading forum for all health services including clinical services. The parties within the forum are now recognised as commissioners of services on behalf of populations, and providers of services who enter into agreements with the commissioners. A good deal of debate has ensued in the literature on health policy as to the exact nature and nomenclature to be used to describe this trading forum. Whilst Enthoven's description of an internal

Strategic Issues in Health Care Management. Edited by M. Malek, J. Rasquinha and P. Vacani
© 1993 John Wiley & Sons Ltd

market has been widely adopted, for the purposes of this paper the elegant usage of the term *quasi-market*, by Le Grand will be used (Le Grand 1989).

A NEW RELATIONSHIP

The medium for the relationship between the provider and the commissioner is the contract. It is both a physical representation and an embodiment of the spirit of the trading agreement between the parties. Furthermore, the contract provides the conduit for communication, information, evaluation, specification and payment for services.

Consequently, what has emerged has been the development of a contractual relationship focused upon buyer and seller roles for the commissioners and the providers. The course and outcome of the contracts can be seen as a function of negotiation in its broadest sense. Whilst the NHS Management Executive issued guidance, together with a model contract for the parties involved (NHS ME 1990), there was no guidance available on how to actually bring the contract about, let alone the importance of negotiation nor the behavioural challenges involved.

It was recognised at an early stage in the development of the quasi-market that there were incentives for both co-operation and conflict between the commissioners and providers, and this prophesying had been further informed by experience in the US health market (Culyer and Posnett 1990). Given such a situation, it was to be expected that much of the negotiation which has occurred is of the mixed-motive type (Walton and McKersie 1966).

It is useful to examine briefly the range of contradictory incentives which are operating in the new systems. It is the commissioners' responsibility to ensure that the health care needs of their own residents are met. There is certainly a widely held belief from the providers' point of view that they should remain as a viable operating unit. The vast majority of providers carry high fixed costs and have developed their provision in response to long standing service patterns. The providers therefore, wish to supply their existing services, but the purchasers may wish to purchase in line with their own medium and long-term policy targets. The sum of these different incentives results in a tension surrounding agreement upon product mix, output rates, unit cost, and agreed definitions or proxies for quality.

NEW EXPERTISE

Drawing on their experience of management expertise in the US health system, Weiner and Ferriss (1990) have emphasised the importance of both managers and clinicians being able to negotiate effectively in the new marketplace. Surprisingly, from the government's point of view, there seems to have been an assumption that managers and clinicians would have acquired these skills during the Resource Management Initiative. Commentators upon the UK experience of the market to date appear to be more optimistic about the abilities of the providers than the purchasers :

It was seen as essential to the success of the market that the health authorities as purchasing agencies should rapidly acquire the confidence, skills and authority to hold their own in their negotiations with the providers. (Butler 1992: 77)

What is now generally recognised in recent negotiation theory is that the view of a negotiator as being only motivated by limited self interest and having no regard for the outcome of the negotiation in terms of the other parties wants and needs is probably going to result in an unsuccessful negotiation in any case. Thus, the Dual Concern Model of Pruitt and Rubin (1986); Blake and Mouton's Conflict Grid (1964); and the Principled Negotiation Approach of Fisher and Ury (1981), have much to offer the commissioners and providers in terms of a learning approach for their negotiations.

THE LEARNING WORKSHOP

An acute hospital, which became an NHS trust in the first wave in 1991 had experienced one round of negotiations with its main purchaser and, as result of this, had identified a number of areas which they wished to explore prior to the next round of negotiations. These were as follows :

- an understanding of the role of the management group in the contract negotiating;
- the opportunity to look at the effect of the contract decisions made by the contracts manager upon the clinical directorates;
- to develop negotiation skills in a learning environment and to further the management development of the whole team including the clinical managers.

To achieve these objectives a learning workshop was devised based upon a simulation of a negotiation between the trust and its major purchaser, which was the local health authority commissioner. The workshop was designed on the basis of an experiential learning style. Such an approach was felt to be appropriate for the group involved, especially as all the clinical directors had taken part in similar training events and were familiar with Kolb's (Kolb 1984) four stage cycle of experiential learning. Furthermore, there is evidence that management development for professionals is enhanced by such an approach (White 1992).

The workshop was run over a period of three days, and it was decided that the group learning would be more effective if the purchasers were not invited to participate. To further learning, it was also decided to use role play, although the risks inherent in such a technique were recognised by the facilitator of the workshop (Van Ments 1983). The two particular variants of role play which were used were, incident play, where parts of the previous negotiation were re-enacted and role reversal. Jaques has demonstrated that such an approach can be particularly useful in interdisciplinary team-work development (Jaques 1986). The workshop also drew upon the experience of the "Rubber Windmill" simulation exercise run by East Anglia

Regional Health Authority, especially in terms of encouraging participants to play out the roles of other professionals, which was often done in a stereotypical manner.

The twenty-three participants in the group were divided into either provider or purchaser roles and each group was given a separate brief, unknown to their counterparts in the other group. The joint constraint upon both groups was that a contract had to be signed within two and half days of the commencement of the simulation, if this did not occur then the exercise would be deemed a failure. The real time corollary of such a failure would result in putting the financial viability of the trust in jeopardy.

Table 1 outlines the range of constraints under which the two parties were required to operate and which were outlined in their briefs. In addition, each party was given a set of common details relating to the contracts — these included details of base and variable prices, the required efficiency savings and settlement arrangements, together with a range of purchaser defined quality standards.

Table 1. Negotiating constraints for purchaser and providers in negotiation simulation

PURCHASERS	PROVIDERS
Information	*Information*
• Future financial year absolute allocation not yet finalised	• Inflation funding of 1% possible for next financial year
• Inflation funding of 1% possible	• Contingency Plans to deal with failure to secure sufficient income to cover all costs had been drafted
	• Pre-committed capital programme summary of end of year contracted activity
	• End of year income summary sheets, by purchaser and contracts
Targets	*Targets*
• To achieve no in-patient waiting lists in any speciality of no longer than 18 months	• Must achieve 1% cost improvement on previous year's allocation (receipts)
• Must obtain a commitment for an extra 4% activity for every 1% extra spent with the Trust	• Must demonstrate 6% target return on capital assets
	• Need to achieve sufficient income to cover variable and fixed costs
Behavioural	*Behavioural*
• Last experience of difficult negotiations with particular individuals	• Past experience of difficult negotiation with particular individuals

Patients' Charter monitoring requirements were also available to each group. A number of service specifications were available for the groups to consult as were some pre-negotiated base line policies and protocols. In effect, these policies, especially the clinical prescribing responsibilities and those relating to the welfare of children and young people in hospital served to act as additional negotiating constraints upon the groups. In short therefore, the participants were working under pressure of time, with constraints they had no control over and with imperfect information. In these respects the simulation mirrored the conditions under which contracts were being negotiated in real time.

CONCEPTS OF NEGOTIATION

Some understanding of negotiation theory is useful to help explain not only the outcome, but also the process by which a negotiation progresses. A theoretical base can also provide a framework for subsequent analysis and prediction. The groups in the simulation exercise had little or no theoretical knowledge, although a number of them were familiar with the popular edition of the Principled Negotiation Approach — 'Getting to Yes' (Fisher and Ury).

There was the danger, especially for the clinical members of the group, of a tendency for requests for a theoretical input into the simulation session from the facilitator. In turn, this was interpreted by the facilitator as a request for a more didactic approach to learning, certainly, a situation, that at least in terms of their professional training the clinicians were more accustomed to. However, it was felt by the team as a whole that the impact of the simulation would be reduced if this had occurred. Consequently, a series of notes were issued about negotiation theory after the workshop. It will inform the subsequent staged analysis of the negotiation if a brief review of some of the theory is presented here.

Three broad categories of negotiation theory can be drawn from the literature, in turn these correspond to a similar categorisation for organisational theory; no doubt because of the roots of empirical negotiation studies in industrial relation settings (Loveridge 1979; Strauss 1978). The first category which can be classified as mechanical or scientific theory, in the tradition of Fayol, which is particularly interested in the legitimisation of power as being singularly a function of organisational position within a hierarchical setting. Whereas, Human Relation or Trait theory, focus upon power being not so much a positional issue, but more a result of relative networks and relationships between individuals, which in turn, helps create informal organisations. Both these groups of theories deal with conflict in terms of an entity which can be eliminated rather than that which is inherently structural to any system.

The behavioural based theories also treat conflict as endemic or prevalent. The difference in their approach is that rather than take the elimination approach, such conflict can be managed, usually by a process of negotiation. The organisational corollary is that organisations then become networks of negotiations. Moreover, this approach allows for the contingent element which is lacking in the mechanical and trait models, for which they have been criticised. A behavioural approach makes an allowance in terms of dealing with peoples' different perceptions of reality, wherein reality itself may become the object of conflict. Much of the contribution towards this approach has come from Rojot (1991), who neatly incorporates the ideas involved in bounded rationality theory with those of negotiation behaviour . Such an approach involves the following assumptions:

i.   behaviour is rational in the eyes of the actor in terms of their own set of objectives, consequently, any behaviour which is exhibited will make sense to the actor in terms of these objectives;
ii.   negotiating parties may not necessarily see negotiating situation in the same way as each other. In turn, this means that they may not have a common definition of what they are actually negotiating nor even why they are negotiating, i.e. they will have different agendas;
iii. the acceptance that people operate within their own bounded rationality and logic, means that reasoning alone will not work to alter or dissuade either party of their position or of the views which they hold.

What benefit is there in understanding this theoretical base in terms of conducting a successful negotiation? The benefits flow from the understanding that if behavioural issues influence an individual's view of the world, then in order to obtain any progress in a negotiation, each party must take cognisance of the other party's desired outcome, not only out of co-operative concern but also for instrumental reasons — for their own success. Hence they will develop a 'win-win' approach and will attempt to bring about some form of mutuality in the negotiation. So, to contextualise some of the theory for application in the purchaser/provider contract negotiation forum, let us look at where the potential for 'dual concern' is available, where the incentives to reach a win-win outcome are, and if we can speculate, what is the bounded rationality of a group of purchasers and providers?

INCENTIVES TO REACH A POSITIVE OUTCOME

The job of the purchasers is to secure health care services on behalf of their population — they are required to do this in the light of the real needs of the population. Albeit, that the very difficulties of defining, let alone measuring need, were not going to be solved by the advent of the reforms. Still, in theory this has meant that they would wish to purchase planned services, rather than services that had been provided as a result of historical utilisation. Thus, their priority setting has to become explicit, and their contracts statements of policy intent.

However, given the situation of a single large provider, it would be possible for them to be in such a dominant position to, whilst not actually preventing, make it very difficult for the achievement of widespread service changes unless it was in their interest to do so. On the other hand, the providers have to ensure their financial viability now that they can no longer rely upon a definite annual budget allocation as a guaranteed source of income, it is in their interest, up to a point, to go along with the demands of the purchaser in order to secure the business. The added problem for the supplier then becomes the need to reconcile the commercial imperative with the desires of clinical autonomy.

Put in these terms it could almost be said that the purchaser and providers have a symbiotic relationship, but such a symbiosis only operates where there is no competition to the single provider. If there are alternative suppliers, then the bargaining power of the purchasers is vastly improved. Similarly, for the provider, an interest in settlement will be sharpened, as will the need to generate alternative sources of income. Competition serves to alter the balance of power between the parties and it is the agreement *up to a point* that is the dynamic for negotiation. It was the purpose of the workshop to test the dynamic and to provide an opportunity to learn about, not only the content of the negotiations, but also the process.

ANALYTICAL FRAMEWORK FOR NEGOTIATION WORKSHOP

The workshop had two facilitators for each group, whose purpose it was to provide process commentary and feedback. The facilitator also had the task of providing the retrospective analysis upon the whole negotiation and to interpret the outcomes in the light of the processes which had occurred. Table 2. shows three possible analytical frameworks for the negotiation process. These are drawn from Pruitt and Carnevale's "Dual Concern Model"; Fisher and Ury's "Principled Negotiation Model" and a synthesis of Rojot's "Analytical Grids" which are used to assess the process of negotiation and the interaction of the negotiators.

Whilst they use different taxonomies, essentially the three frameworks demonstrate that any negotiation will be concerned with a problem or issue; it will involve people in relation to others and will occur within an environment which itself will provide opportunities or constraints. These three factors will then result in variations in bargaining power. The negotiation can also be analysed in terms of distinct phases through an opening position to a collective middle position and onto an eventual agreement and implementation, or failure and withdrawal from the negotiation. Within the negotiation therefore, there are both substantive issues to be agreed, together with procedures and relationships to be dealt with, all of which in themselves may become a point of negotiation.

The workshop was not videoed but the facilitators used the framework in table 2. to keep a record of activities, together with details of speech and behaviour. The participants kept a record of options, offers, agreements and data. The same framework was used to provide the retrospective process commentary in the feedback session and is used here to present an analysis of the negotiation simulation and its outcome.

ANALYSIS OF NEGOTIATION WORKSHOP

Opening Stage

The two groups, acting as purchasers and providers, chose to start the exercise with the selection of a negotiating team of four people each. The two teams then chose to

Table 2. Analytical framework for negotiation simulation feedback

Common Generic Factors	Fisher & Ury	Rojot	Pruitt & Carnevalle
Topic under consideration. Substantive interests	*The problem* —"don't bargain over positions"	*The negotiating item.* *Mixed items.* — distributive — integrative	*Issues / options / divergence of interests*
Relational	*The people*	*The parties and their relationship* — degree of permanence of the relationship — attitudes to each other	*Relationships among the negotiating parties* — power — trust
Environment	*Resources / Constraints / Time / Social Norms*		
Relative bargaining power	*Function of:*	— *people / parties* — *environment* — *objectives*	
The Process ➔	*Focus on interests, not on positions*	*Expression of collective rationalities*	*Expression of dual concern & problem solving*

⬇   ⬇   ⬇   ⬇

- Procedural Rules - meetings/rooms/seating
- Collection and exchange of information
- Use of common criteria
- Use of representative
- Use of third party
- Use of mediator
- Adjournments

Behaviour ➔

- Communication
- Non-verbal communication
- Recording
- Emotions
- Symbolism
- Use of tactics
- Mediation

Stages and Phases ➔ OPENING

- diagnosis
- judgement
- prescription
- deadlock/conflict

MIDDLE

- broadening options
- brainstorming
- proposals/counter proposals
- information exchange
- joint definitions of potential agreement
- 'what if' scenarios

CONCLUDING PHASE & OUTCOME

- clear statement of agreement
- clarification of detail and technicalities
- agreement on commitment
- discussion of implementation

meet in one room, which became known as the negotiating room whilst the remainder of the groups acted as an audience to the negotiation. When active inter-team negotiation was not occurring, each group retired to a separate room which became known as the briefing rooms. Thus, very early on in the exercise both inter- and intra-group territory was established. In turn, this territory was functionally defined in terms of negotiating and briefing. The pattern was retained for the whole exercise, as was the team negotiating approach, although the team members did change at a later stage. Some neutral ground was also established informally and this tended to be in the corridor and circulation space. No specific request for recording the proceedings was made although within the groups some members did take personal notes.

There was an early agreement upon timing, structure and schedule of meetings. Again, this was kept to throughout the whole period. In terms of room settings and seating arrangements, the teams adopted a meetings approach with members facing each other over a set of tables in a formal, almost confrontational manner, delineated in terms of 'us' and 'them'. Each team had a leader, a main spokesperson, and two support people, one of whom adopted the role of clinical expert.

The dialogue between the two teams began with an exchange of information relating to the activity levels experienced at the Trust in relation to the agreed contract levels with the purchaser. There was no agreement upon this particular issue until six hours before the end of the simulation. Without agreement upon the previous year's out-turn it was not possible to agree a baseline position for the new financial year. After the first failure to agree these figures the teams adjourned. Throughout the whole exercise adjournments were used, either tactically or for when the teams wished to consult with their group members.

Middle Stage

After a number of abortive attempts to agree figures, the purchasers tabled their list of objectives. These were clearly stated in terms of their purchasing intentions as follows:

- a large increase in the number of day case procedures across all specialities;
- dramatic reductions for inpatient and outpatient waiting lists, beyond those of the Patients Charter targets;
- a four percent increase in activity in each contract category with a one percent increase in contract cost;
- targeted developments for certain specialties especially the elderly and any development which was in accordance with *Health of The Nation* targets.

From this point on in the negotiation the purchasers took the initiative. Consequently, the rest of the exercise was spent in negotiating those topics where the provider was placed on the defensive. All their group meetings were spent working out whether it was operationally possible to deliver the purchaser requirements.

Never in the course of the simulation did the provider have, or make, the opportunity to place their own agenda on the table. Meanwhile, in the 'corridor' the financial and activity positions were being clarified and options for a way forward suggested by the two financial representatives.

At this point in the process the provider changed their team to include a clinical representative from each of the specialties under discussion, when it was being assessed as to whether the waiting list reductions were achievable. It was at this stage that the differences in the briefing room activities began to show. The purchasers now began to wait for a reply from the providers and the atmosphere was relaxed and confident. On the other hand in the provider's room the internal negotiation had begun between the clinicians and the general managers of the Trust. There was evidence of internal tension in that the provider's business plan had included a number of capital developments for services which had not been included in the purchasers target groups for service growth. Above all, there was serious doubt amongst the clinicians that they could achieve the levels of day case procedures being requested with the equipment and technology currently available to them in the hospital.

As a result of the internal provider negotiations the main negotiation recommenced with a number of counter proposals from the providers. These related to the numbers of day cases it was possible to perform and the waiting list times. After a joint exercise in developing operationally achievable targets, a draft outline was agreed between the parties. However, the purchasers were unwilling to give any concessions in respect of the volume increases which they expected and the additional financing for this. Another lengthy adjournment followed in which the majority of the activity came from the providers briefing room.

Concluding Phase

With only two hours to go before the contract signing deadline, the two groups could not reach agreement. At this stage the team members had completely changed to include the members of all the actual contracting team — the chief executive, the contracts manager and the medical director — with no other clinical representatives. The time prior to the final meeting had again been taken up with internal provider negotiations. This time they focused on the financial effects of having to do more work for less money. The only option available to them was to re-asses their cost improvement programmes and to increase their targets in respect of their income generation programme. Once this had been agreed the two teams were able to sign the contract, but it was the purchaser who felt that they had a successful outcome. As far as the provider was concerned they only felt that it could have been "much worse".

Observations of behaviour amongst the two groups showed similar patterns of frustration, anger, sarcasm and tiredness. The effort involved in the negotiation process was a surprise to some members and a high level of visible emotion was evident. Non-verbal communication showed signs of poor listening and disagreement between the groups. However, intra-group support was strong and there was always reference to corporate objectives and values with many members referring to the statements made in the Trust's business plan.

COMMENTARY OF THE NEGOTIATION PROCESS & OUTCOME

The actual negotiation was not a successful one in terms of a win-win outcome. Both groups adopted the positional bargaining approach; there was little evidence of high 'other concern'. Not once was there an attempt to establish a joint agenda nor to understand the other party's negotiating reality and rationality. One of the most telling comments came from a team member during the plenary session when he said that: "...we should have had talks about talks".

Whilst a simulation can never truly represent the real time negotiation, those people who were normally involved in the process did comment upon how realistic the event was. This was especially so in terms of the time constraints. The people who perform the Trust's negotiations also have operational responsibilities whereas the purchasers appear to have more time in which to negotiate. They also have the strongest bargaining position as they have the money, and thus the initiative will always lie with them. The provider was in a stronger position in terms of access to information and to be able to verify data. The provider is currently at an advantage because of their involvement in the resource management initiative, but this is likely to be only temporary.

WHAT LESSONS WERE LEARNT?

The simulation proved to be a learning experience at two levels: First, in terms of the Trust's approach to negotiation; Secondly, it also has a broader application to contract negotiation in the quasi-market in general.

Lessons for the Trust

The Trust realised that it should have started the process of negotiation earlier, and made attempts to agree a joint agenda with the purchaser. The experience of the workshop also showed them that success involved managerial commitment and continuity and that internal communication was vital.

All involved realised that agreements made at the negotiating table must be operationally feasible. Some negotiation will be on an expert-to-expert basis. Business planning in isolation is not helpful, it also needs to be done in the light of the major purchaser's strategy. There was a tendency to accept that some extra work could be taken on at marginal cost to the Trust, this may prove to not always be the case, and volume decisions need to be backed with financial information.

The most important information for making product-mix decisions was the case-mix information which should be available in such a way as to facilitate easy modelling on a 'what if' basis to support negotiating options. Much more summary information was needed in a form understandable to all parties. If a financial penalty system was introduced, especially for guaranteed waiting list times, it was felt that the agreements would be more binding.

General Lessons

There is the likelihood that the negotiating forum will become a policy making forum, or at least the forum wherein policy is conveyed to the provider. If this should become the case then not only does it add more agenda items to the negotiation process, it also means that added pressure is brought to bear on the provider in terms of the need to model the financial and operational effects of such policies.

The process did demonstrate a considerable change in the relationship between the two parties. In some places this will be more marked because of the previous executive role of the DHAs whose personnel may be members of the negotiation team. Managerial and commercial expertise appears to be on the side of the providers, however, this new found confidence and independence was constrained by the sapiential authority of the purchasers who were acting as the voice of government in terms of securing policy objectives through contracts.

There was no recourse to a third party, or mediator, in fact each of the two groups agreed that they would rather operate within a series of compromises rather than refer to the NHS Management Executive outpost. Such behaviour raises the interesting point of regulation: there appeared to be evidence of a desire for self regulation and to limit the involvement of others in the contract settlement.

For the senior executives who are going to negotiate there is likely to be a need for more rather than less detail, this is especially so in terms of a knowledge of their unit's performance. In turn, this could lead to even more overloading and conflict of priorities.

There is evidence of purchasing consortia forming and this will serve to increase the sophistication of information requirements which may not be matched at provider level, hence causing more difficulty in reconciling base data to commence the negotiations with. The role of an effective negotiating leader will become an imperative. In many cases this task will fall to the contracts manager. However, in the final stages of the negotiation it is highly probable that the chief executives will become involved, not least because they will than have the task of obtaining commitment from the operating units - or clinical directorates. Thus, the person specification for such jobs will in the future need to include negotiation skills.

CONCLUDING COMMENTS

The current lack of procedural guidelines for contract negotiation in the NHS has meant that a number of purchaser and providers are learning the skills and acquiring an understanding of negotiation as they go along. A negotiation simulation workshop provides a safe learning environment to develop these skills. It also proved to be particularly useful in terms of introducing those clinicians who would not normally be involved in the negotiation process to the problems of reaching an agreement. Similarly, it helped demonstrate the need for contracts managers to communicate with clinicians before agreeing to demanding performance targets which may not be operationally or technically feasible.

The author was also particularly interested in what was not negotiated in the workshop. Such issues were the transaction costs of the contracting process; more detailed deliberation upon price as opposed to access and volume; the use of comprehensive clinical audit to support assertions of quality and the failure to discuss a joint strategy-making forum between purchasers and providers. It is felt that these areas offer a fertile ground for further research.

REFERENCES

Appleby, J., Middlemas, K. and Ranade, W., (1989), "Provider markets: a glimpse of the future". Health Service Journal, 99, 414-15. Blake, R. R. and Mouton, J. S., (1964), The Managerial Grid, Gulf Press, Houston.

Butler, J., (1992), Patients, Policies and Politics: Before and After Working for Patients, Open University Press, Buckingham.

Culyer, A. J. and Posnett, J., (1990), "Hospital Behaviour and Competition", Culyer, A. J., Maynard, A. K. and Posnett, J.W (eds), Competition in Health care: Reforming the NHS, Macmillan, Basingstoke, 12-48.

Fisher, R. and Ury, W., (1981) Getting to YES: Negotiating agreement without giving in. Houghton Mifflin, Boston.

Jaques, D., (1986), Training for Teamwork - Report of the Thamesmead Interdisciplinary Project, Oxford Polytechnic, Educational Methods Unit, Oxford.

Kolb, D. A., (1984), Experiential Learning, Prentice Hall, Englewood Cliffs, New Jersey.

Le Grand, J., (1990) Quasi - markets and Social policy, School of Advanced Urban Studies, University of Bristol, Studies in Decentralisation and Quasi - Markets, No. 1

Loveridge, R. and Egan, W., (1979), Notes on the theory and techniques of negotiation, unpublished, Aston University Business School.

National Health Service Management Executive (1990), Contracts for Health Services: Operating Contracts, London, HMSO.

Pruitt, D. G. and Rubin, J. Z., (1986), Social Conflict: Escalation, stalemate, and settlement. Mc Graw - Hill, New York.

Pruitt, D G. and Carnevale, P J., (1993), Negotiation In Social Conflict, Open University Press., Buckingham.

Rojot, J., (1991), Negotiation: From Theory to Practice, Macmillan Basingstoke.

Strauss, A., (1978), Negotiations: Varieties, Contexts, Processes and Social Order, Jossey - Bass, San Francisco.

Van Ments, M., (1983), Effective Use of Role Play, Kogan Page, London.

Walton, R. E. and McKersie, R. B., (1966), "Behavioural dilemmas in mixed - motive decision making", Behavioural Science, 11, Sept. 370-384.

Weiner, J. P. and Ferriss, D. M., (1990) GP Budget Holding in the UK: Lessons From America. Research Report No. 7, King's Fund Institute, London.

White, J. A., (1992), "Applying an Experiential Learning Styles Framework to Management and Professional Development", Journal of Management Development, 11(5), 55-64.

Willcocks, A. J., (1967), The Creation of the National Health Service, London, Routledge and Kegan Paul.

23 Strategic Issues in Municipal Services for Community Prevention in the Netherlands

ANDRE W.M. MEIJER

Rijksuniversiteit Limburg, The Netherlands

INTRODUCTION

Making strategic choices to gain sufficient legitimacy and other resources, is nowadays a major problem for the management of most local or district public health services for community health protection, prevention and promotion (community prevention) in the Netherlands. For these (former) municipal health departments — in Holland known as 'Gemeentelijke Gezondheidsdiensten' (GGDs) face at the moment many inconsistent or even conflicting external and internal norms and demands.

At the present time a GGD is expected to implement new health policies which are formulated at the national level. At the same time a GGD has to prepare and execute health policies and programmes at the local or district level. In this second role a GGD has to reflect the political visions, conflicts and decisions to gain legitimacy. But a GGD is not only an instrument of another organization but also an organization in itself.

Being a department of the municipal bureaucracy, a GGD has its own structure, rules and interests. But as a professional service organization for health care and community prevention on the other hand, a GGD has its own professional standards and strivings. To keep the balance between these positions (and roles) is 'sometimes a hell of a job' for the management of a GGD.

Thus a central research question is: how do GGD-managers satisfy inconsistent environmental and internal norms and produce co-ordinated organizational action simultaneously ?

In the following sections a short overview of the development and organization of local and district public health services for community prevention in the Netherlands is given. Attention is also focused on some recent organizational and management problems with respect to GGDs. The paper ends with a case illustration of the phenomena under study and draw some conclusions.

Strategic Issues in Health Care Management. Edited by M. Malek, J. Rasquinha and P. Vacani
© 1993 John Wiley & Sons Ltd

OVERVIEW OF THE SECTOR

In the course of time a diversity of mainly not-for-profit organizations, publicly as well as privately owned, at the national as well as at the local level, are involved in 'community prevention' in the Netherlands. The biggest organization among these is the State Institute for Public Health and Environmental Protection (RIVM), mainly a research institute. Much better known to the public are the 62 GGDs, the health departments of the municipalities, functioning as public services for community prevention at the local or district level.

The GGD of Amsterdam is the biggest with a staff of 860 FTE for about 710,000 inhabitants and a budget of Dfl. 87 million. The smallest GGD has a staff of 20 FTE for almost 50,000 inhabitants (Meijer 1991; Timmers 1991).

Whereas the newest GGD dates from January 1990, the oldest GGD was founded in Amsterdam in March 1893. About 20 GGDs followed in the first three decades of this century. These first GGDs started as organizations for primary prevention. The greatest health problems of that time were related to medical-technical (i.e. technical-hygienic) problems: bad living and working conditions, especially in the overcrowded cities. For this reason most activities at that time were directed at examinations into the health status of the population (community diagnosis) and the implementation of measures against infectious diseases in daily living life.

The development of GGDs in the following decades saw a constant process of growth and expansion, and of task differentiation and specialisation. Such development was caused and facilitated by the rapid developments in technological solutions for the biggest health problems of the era and by political changes in the city councils. Many independent public installations and services, such as sanitary sewage disposal, water purification and supply, refuse collection, house and building inspection, working place inspection, food inspection, and can be traced back to the activities and the knowledge of these municipal health departments (De Swaan 1989; Meijer 1991).

Since then the GGDs have concentrated their attention more and more on social-medical (i.e. medical-hygienic) problems, with an orientation on disease as a disfunctioning aspect of the biophysical human system of individuals[1]. Secondary prevention such as planning and executing programmes for health surveillance of risk groups like school-age children, early diagnosis of specific diseases (screening and case-finding), infection control, immunization against infectious or communicable diseases, and prevention of sexually transmittable diseases, as well as activities for preventive dental care for the youth, became the core activities of the GGDs. Besides these tasks most GGDs are now performing advisory roles in the field of social security and social services (advice to individuals), of occupational health for employees in the public sector, and of hygiene inspection of schools, camping sites, swimming pools and other public places and buildings as well. Most GGDs also

---

[1]One may speak of a double reduction process in prevention: from a holistic-ecological approach to a medical-hygienistic approach, and from a society-oriented to an individual-oriented approach of health (or sickness).

have tasks in the field of medical and paramedical first aid and assistance in case of calamities, of (emergent) ambulance services, and of assistance services for drug abuse.

From 1974 to 1990 the Dutch national government has stimulated further development of community prevention (primary and secondary prevention). Greater attention is paid to the multi-dimensionality of health, to inequalities in health, to the different determinants of health and diseases (like lifestyles and the social and physical environment). Epidemiological analyses of populations and health diagnoses of environments are the best tools for research in this field. Special attention has to be paid to health surveillance and the execution of prevention programmes for groups with great(er) health risks, to the prevention and control of contagious diseases, and to the promotion and education of healthier behaviour of the population in general, especially the young. Progress in community health has to be realised by means of policy making and implementation within communities, in connection with inter-sectoral co-operation and with community participation, all under the responsibility of the municipality. Since then the professional societies, the National Associations of Municipalities (VNG) and the association of GGDs are paying much more attention to the development of new ways of health promotion and health protection (see De Leeuw 1989; De Leeuw *et al* 1991). In connection with the WHO-Europe, the 'Healthy Cities' project has been started (Van der West *et al* 1992). One really can speak of 'a renaissance of public health' (Crown, 1989), or 'the dawn of a new public health policy' (Kaasjager et al 1987).

A second national goal since 1974 has been the formation of a nation-wide, closed network of public local or district services with similar goals and tasks with regard to the new formulated community prevention. From 1985 to 1989 special financial stimulation was being given to speed up this process.

THE SUCCESS OF CENTRAL GOVERNMENT POLICY

Government policy has first resulted in a new legislation of community prevention, called 'Wet Collectieve Preventie Volksgezondheid' or 'WCPV' (1990). The statutory task of all municipalities at present is to assume responsibility for the health of the population by taking care of community prevention activities at the local or district level. This has to be done through the development and the co-ordination of programmes and actions aimed at guarding, maintaining and improving the health of all inhabitants. To accomplish these prevention tasks (development, co-ordination and often the execution of prevention programmes), a municipality has to maintain, alone or with other municipalities, a public service organization for community prevention — the GGD. But beside the requirement for a GGD for every municipality, the municipalities determine the tasks and job descriptions of the local (or district) GGD. A municipality is, moreover, autonomous in spending a certain amount of tax-money on the GGD. A municipality alone, or together with others, is also independent in putting forward norms or standards to measure the functioning, products (services) and effects of a GGD with respect to the tasks of the GGD in general and the attention paid to community prevention in particular.

Secondly, the Green Papers on community prevention, temporary financial support, and the new act, resulted directly in the formal creation of the few 'missing' GGDs. The national and professional policies, the subsidies and the new legislation also caused the reconstruction of many 'old' municipal health departments into 'modern' GGDs. A nation-wide network of 62 public organizations for modern community prevention services, on behalf of about 600 municipalities has now been completed[2]. This can be considered as 'the completion of the first building phase' (Van de Water 1989: 6) or of 'the achievement of a certain stage in the institutionalisation of a (sub)sector in society'. This process of institutionalisation of a societal sub-sector exists of three partial processes: a normative process of articulation and objectification of values, a functional process of structuring, and a political process of mobilisation and stabilisation (Eisenstadt 1968; Peper 1972; Meijer 1993a)[3].

CURRENT POSITIONS AND ROLES OF A GGD

With respect to national health policies formulated by Parliament and the Ministry of Health, a municipality and its GGD are seen as instruments for the implementation of those policies. In this light the national government holds the position of the political and administrative principal, and the municipalities and the GGDs are their agents. It is the GGDs role to execute such national policies. However, government policies are bound to be general in character. This is all the more the case with respect to the (re)formulated paradigm on community health ('Health for all'). This ambiguity is almost unavoidable, leading to re-interpretations of those policies by municipalities and GGDs during the implementation process. Those who implement government policies have values of their own and will give meaning they prefer to the policies (Lincoln 1985). This results in processes of mutual adjustment and co-optation (Berman and McLaughlin, 1976)[4]. The consequences a GGD has to deal with are new ambiguity and conflicts at the local level. So this agency position and executive role, in combination with the new broad health policy and legislation, are leading to new, often inconsistent institutional norms and external demands for municipalities and the GGDs.

At the local or district level a GGD is, again, formally an instrument (or agency) for 'independent' health policy making and implementation. But, as a part of the public administration at this level a GGD has not only to follow but also to guide its own municipal council(s). As a department with special expertise it plays its own

---

[2]In organizational terms, the set of GGDs is not a network but an association (or population) of organizations.

[3]Another part of this research project, completed in concept, is a description and analysis of the institutionalisation of public services for community prevention in the Netherlands on the sector level.

[4]Both can be found as we have discovered in our research (Meijer 1993a).

roles (and games) within the political and administrative organization and processes. When the professional staff of a GGD take, for example, the side of a complaining group of inhabitants, this coalition may take over the power of the politicians. Politicians who play the objective role in that case risking making themselves redundant (Brunsson 1989: 63-64). So a GGD is potentially an influential actor with respect to local health policy making and implementation.

In most cities and districts, however, GGDs are not interested in politics. As a professional public service with tasks and activities in the field of secondary prevention, most GGDs have been living in splendid isolation during the last decades. Many city councils have seen the GGD as a subsidized private organisation and not as a municipal health department. But the recent differentiation and explicit formulation of old and new tasks, and above all the changes in financing rules have activated the local politicians and city managers, and, in the case of a district GGD, also the members of the board and commissions of the district GGDs. Politicians see new problems and solutions and city managers want greater value for public money. Processes of politicisation and rationalization of the GGD have occurred. Additionally, power conflicts between administrations of different municipalities have existed for a long time and in relation to a broad range of topics. Health has become a new subject of district conflicts. So the GGD is becoming a player in the arena of a party political or city and district administrative conflicts[5].

As an organization for public health services, a GGD is a department of the municipal administration and also a professional health care organization. In the past splendid isolation some GGDs have developed into more professional health care services. They developed an independent position to comply with a broad range of old and new specific professional or technical norms and standards. Some others have developed into more bureaucratic organizations with their own specific characteristics. Some GGDs have become an 'institution' in themselves, with their own rules and values; a committed polity, with a clear identity and purpose, serving the selfish strivings of its participants (Perrow 1986: 168). Existing GGDs have their own history and identity which will not be changed in a short period of time or even can not be changed at all. This means that new external influences may lead to different reactions. Professional conflicts may arise.

But also other issues have arisen. In the first place a GGD has to fulfil 'old' tasks. This concerns, in particular, routine practices like screening populations and medical examinations of individuals, and other fields, like occupational health and ambulance services, where substitution exists (or may arise) and a price mechanism may work. It is sure that the municipalities expect their GGDs to accomplish these tasks as professionally and efficiently as possible. Also, the municipalities seek more and more value for money. So a GGD is ever increasingly working in a transactional environment or in a (quasi) market.

---

[5]The biggest health problems often only concern the biggest city or cities but not the smaller municipalities. So the last don't want to take responsibility for problems of others and, above all, they don't want to pay for the solution(s) of the problems of others.

Alternatively, as an organization for the newly reformulated community prevention, a GGD works mainly in that part of the health field that can be characterized by the absence of spontaneous client or market demand. Here little market incentive or market regulation exist. These new tasks, up to now, have been based on an abstract ideology and a vague mission (i.e. health for all through community prevention), broad formulated goals (prolonging life and preventing illness of risk groups), more or less weak technologies with unclear indicators for performance or product-output (health promotion, health education, health policy making, promoting health in other public policies etc), and little tangible evidence of the impact of such activities (gain of health of the population). There are even no statutory indications of minimum resource-capacities in terms of money, or staff, to be spent by municipalities on these specific prevention tasks. Therefore, with respect to these new tasks, a GGD faces mainly institutional norms as indicators for performance, enforced by new legislation, by new and expected municipal health policies, by some vague professional standards or by reflection of old traditions. In this sense a GGD has to live in an institutional environment — although in this field more and more market-like, transactional norms arise (Meijer 1993a). Because these new policies and tasks are ambiguous, they are susceptible to political and administrative conflicts. They also may conflict with the views of more traditional professional (or bureaucratic) groups inside a GGD.

To sum up, many a contemporary GGD needs to adopt multiple positions and to perform many roles with respect to a mixture of more or less independent job responsibilities. It also performs a very mixed range of tasks and activities for different kinds of products and services, and with different effects for different groups of customers.

This mixed range of old and new tasks and activities has no fixed order in terms of societal or political problem solving priorities, nor in terms of political, technological or professional standards, nor administrative or market priorities. Also, it is almost completely bound to its municipality or municipalities for resources (legitimacy and money). So the task environment (Thompson 1967) of most GGDs has become much more complex and fragmented than previously.

GGDs face new and old external and internal, transactional and institutional norms and demands, sometimes with no relationship with public health and community prevention. Such norms and demands can be inconsistent and may lead to conflicts between participating groups at the local level. They also may conflict with professional and bureaucratic groups inside the GGD. In order to gain sufficient resources a GGD has to cope with this mixture of external and internal norms and requisites with only one characteristic in common: their relationship with public health and public administration. It is the task of the management, the board and the general management of a GGD to tackle these new strategic issues.

MANAGEMENT TASKS

A natural major task for the management of a GGD is to co-ordinate and integrate the great diversity of activities within the GGD. This mixture of tasks and activities, and the different kinds of external (resource) dependencies, needs a complex mixture of criteria and processes to make the required strategic choices, to allocate the resources, to structure the organization and to control activities and the use of resources (see Goold and Quinn 1990; Hofstede 1981). In this sense a GGD needs to become a more rational, action oriented organization, and also more dependent than before on a changing and sometimes highly political environment from which to seek its necessary resources (legitimacy and money).

Additionally, a GGD has come more and more under the pressure of differing external influences. GGDs have to become more open organizations, more directed and subordinated to municipal politics and administration, especially since that municipality is also the main financier of the GGD. As a consequence the management of a GGD has the task of taking care of most external relations, especially the relations with the participating municipality and the different groups inside those municipalities. A GGD has to become a more political, relation-oriented organization, dependent on its own identity, vision and strategic and tactical behaviour if it wishes to play a role in that field.

So the management has to satisfy the inconsistent environmental, and internal, institutional and transactional norms and to produce co-ordinated organizational action simultaneously to gain needed resources.

In the literature many instruments, strategies and tactics of 'coping with' or 'intervening in' external demands and norms are offered (see: Thompson 1967; Meyer and Rowan 1977; Scott 1987 1992; Harrison 1989;). The institutional, and political, perspective of organizations, put forward by writers such as Meyer and Rowan (1977), Pfeffer (1981, 1992), Meyer and Scott (1983), Scott (1987), Zucker (1988) or Brunsson (1989), and reproduced by others (see Scott (1992), and Reed (1992)), suggest that (the management of) organizations in situations like this might choose, or is forced to choose, between separation of politics and action; and also for strategies and tactics like categorical conformity, structural isomorphism, bridging and buffering relations, and loose coupling of activities, instead of co-ordinating action to produce certain products or services.

The following section expands on the separation of municipal politics and organizational action. The function of decision making is crucial (Brunsson 1989). Decisions are fundamental to all organizations for the adaptation and implementation of talk and discussion into action. Decisions are fundamental to political organizations to demonstrate responsibility and power. Decisions, clarify who formally lead and who are led. In this sense decisions have the function to unite talk and action. But in political organizations decisions demonstrate more the formal possibility of influencing action, than any real influence on the implementation of those decisions.

Decisions are also crucial for action-oriented organizations, not to demonstrate, but to allocate responsibility and power over co-ordinated action. Decisions in action-oriented organizations demonstrate real influence on action. In this sense decisions have the function to separate talk and actions.

GGDs — BETWEEN POLITICS AND ACTION

In an intriguing book on the organization of hypocrisy, Brunsson (1989) made a distinction between two ideal types of organization: one which relies on organized action for ensuring the support of the environment, and one whose legitimacy is based upon its reflection of, sometimes inconsistent, norms in the environment. The first type of organization calls for co-ordination, integration and uniformity of activities to gain legitimacy. Those qualities will imbue organizational structures, processes and outputs, which in turn will achieve maximum efficiency and effectiveness. In the second type of organization, the reflection of inconsistencies calls for politics, for dissolution, disintegration, isolation and a variety in structures, processes and outputs. If one could create, manage and work in organizations which legitimized themselves exclusively, either by politics or by action, it would in a certain sense be simple: each base has its own fairly special clear-cut requirements as regards organizational structure and processes (Brunsson 1989). But many organizations need (or have got) a double basis for legitimacy and survival. If they try to satisfy one legitimation base, they will mismanage the other. So many organizations need this double basis and this presents them with a dilemma.

For example, a municipality is not only a political platform which has to demonstrate political party conflicts to gain political support from voters for another four years; it is also expected to build houses, to construct streets and bridges, or to deliver unpolluted water or first aid in case of emergencies. So for many organizations this dilemma is even 'an insoluble problem' (Brunsson 1989: 33). A choice for one base dissolutes the other.

As a part of a municipality the GGDs also has this double orientation. They have to reflect their discordant political environment because they are required by statute to be a part of the local or district political scene for health policy making and implementation. But also, as professional and public services organizations, GGDs are expected to act orderly and efficiently. These expectations are not only present among the public or the tax-money spending municipalities, but also among their own employees. Thus, as a part of the local or district political platform, GGDs are seen as agents, as instruments for policy making, with little autonomy or freedom to make decisions and decide action. Most politicians expect GGDs to behave and operate in such a manner. But as professional bureaucratic organizations, GGDs try to gain as much autonomy over their scarce resources and their own decisions, actions and performance, as possible.

The basic method for dealing with these conflicting demands is to isolate politics and action, i.e. to decouple them (Weick 1969); see also: Thompson, (1967); Meyer and Rowan, (1977); and Scott (1992). Brunsson indicates that there are four ways in which organizations can separate action from politics: chronologically; by subject matter; in different environments; and in different organizational units (Brunsson,

1989). These four ways of separating politics from action are not mutually exclusive. Most organizations use more than one method. These are now discussed.

Separation of politics and action in time

The separation of politics and action in time means the organization responds to the demands for politics at certain periods and to the demands of action at others. During the political periods the organization becomes an arena for the public demonstration of conflict between individuals, parties or groups. It is important to discuss problems at this period, not solutions. But the ability to produce co-ordinated action is slight. Talk, discussion and political decisions replace action.

At other times the organization responds to demands for action. Disagreement is repressed if it threatens to interfere with organizational action. The organization tries to reach and maintain a consistent common ideology. The organization seeks solutions and actions, not visions, talk, discussion and political decisions. It becomes good at taking action, but bad at reflecting inconsistencies.

Separation of politics and action by topic

Politics and action can also be separated into different topics or issues. While some issues can be used for conducting politics, such as redistribution or subsidy questions, others lend themselves to a stronger action orientation, to attempt to produce action, like highly technical or professional topics. Healthy city policy questions or problems like inequality of health can easily give rise to strong ideological talk and discussions but also seriously jeopardize the chance of realizing any plan or action. For action groups (or private organizations) it is much easier to produce action than for municipalities. But action groups can not survive long or strong ideological discussions as municipalities can.

Separation of politics and action by environments

The organization can also opt for politics or action, depending on the environment with which it is interacting. It can create environments for conducting politics and for producing action.

Separation of politics and action by organizational units

The last option according, to Brunsson, for separating and action is that some units can respond to political demands, and are organized to reflect those political requirements, while other units can respond to demands for action and are organized in a corresponding way. The distinction between a political council and an administrative, functional, organization reflects such a separation by units. But the political and administrative dichotomy becomes more problematic if the organization tries to link the political and administrative sub-organizations together, i.e. if the decisions of the political units are to be made consistent with the decisions and actions of the action unit, or vice versa (Brunsson 1989: 37). And that is just what is happening now in the Netherlands. There is a general striving to conduct politics in a no-nonsense way, to conduct politics like a business firm, on the one hand, and also to politicize the municipalities and the GGD with respect to public health.

A case as illustration

This section examines how managers of GGDs satisfy inconsistent environmental political norms, and simultaneously, produce co-ordinated action to legitimate their organization. A summarisation is given of the way one GGDs managers attempt to achieve this. This is based on policy documents of the GGD, and on interviews with participants in and around it (Meijer 1993b). Our on-going investigations are seeking to obtain complete pictures of the strategic choices and behaviour of GGDs, not for reasons of statistical generalisation but for theoretical generalization and to gain practical insight.

The GGD of Hillcounty[6]

The GGD of Hillcounty was founded by a bigger, central city and taken over by a small number of other municipalities some 15 years ago. The district GGD has a staffing of 110 FTE, serving a population of approximately 180,000 inhabitants. After a long period of tranquillity, isolation and prosperity, this professional, social-medical oriented organization with more or less autonomous sub-departments for mainly medical-hygienic secondary prevention, occupational health services for civil servants and ambulance services, had to face disturbance, outside interference and scarcity. At least three factors have caused great changes in the position and relationships of this organization over the last five years.

Firstly, the general striving of all municipalities in the Netherlands during the eighties to cut costs and to obtain better value for money from all municipal departments, district departments and services. In Hillcounty this initiated discussions in the board of the district GGD on its supposed efficiency and effectiveness, primarily addressing terms of concentration on statutory tasks and agreements on production volumes for the participating municipalities of the district GGD and followed by the question whether to re-organise or even to privatize the district GGD. The board held no discussion on non-statutory tasks nor on the impact (transitive goals in terms of gain of health) of the GGD at all. The board took a position as a client, not as a participant or, let alone, as the leader of this organization, more as stockholders or stakeholders (Meijer 1991). There was an unspoken understanding not to politicize the organization externally or internally with discussions on tasks or ideology. So the board and the staff of the GGD acted like an action oriented organization and wished to continue as such.

The second factor was the wish of the biggest municipality to pay more attention to community prevention in the central city in relation to a national discussion on the

---

[6]This is a fictitious name for an existing GGD.

need for 'social renewal' at the end of the eighties and the new legislation on community prevention (the 'WCPV' of 1990).

The politicians and bureaucrats in the town-hall of the central city realised they had a district health department to give them support on policy making and implementation and to comply with the new law on community prevention. But many of these politicians and bureaucrats hesitated at the same time to discuss these subjects at meetings of the board of the district GGD. They were aware that the other, surrounding villages had never been interested in more central city influence, fearing for their own political and financial independency. They also knew that the major part of the staff of the district GGD was professionally oriented on secondary prevention and not on 'social renewal'; on screening and not on analyses in the field of multiple determinants of the health of (deprived city) populations; and on vaccinating and not on policy making, health promotion and education or interventions with regard to those vague and political 'health ideologies' such as "Health for all by the year 2000". So these politicians and bureaucrats of the central city expected to start conflicts and to lose control if they would drop this topic at the level of the district GGD, as long as they could not change their relations with the GGD and/or influence the policy of this GGD fundamentally. These things became possible by the succession of the CEO of the GGD in 1988 and took place definitely with the modification of the financing regulations in 1990. Until 1990 the GGD was accredited for many of the activities in the field of secondary prevention and thereby partly but directly financed with ear-marked money by the Ministry of Health. But from 1990 on, a municipality alone, or with others, is made totally responsible for the financing of the GGD. So every municipality can fully act as a purchaser of 'GGD-services' and seek for 'value for money'. This changed the independency of the GGD on the municipalities dramatically.

The third group of factors causing change, was related to the succession of the medical director of the GGD in 1988[7]. The new CEO was also trained in medicine, but much younger and more 'open minded'. He wished to establish and strengthen his role and position inside the organization from the very beginning. He took firm decisions on the structure of the organization, in general, and on the tasks and the responsibilities of the professionals and the other leading staff in particular. Advised by an experienced management consultant, he also carefully avoided causing too strong opposition against his decisions and against himself. He feared this would harm the functioning of the organization in the district and/or his career and position as a CEO in the eyes of the board. His ultimate goal was, as he said, to make the organization more efficient and effective. He considered the best way to achieve this was to integrate the different parts and activities of the organization by means of a

---

[7]Other specific reasons are related to some smaller topics with respect to public health and social care, supported by an alderman and a civil servant of the central city. In the administration of the central city exists bureaucratic opposition against 'these kind of loose political projects'. The new CEO of the district GGD accepted these projects with both hands for the desired growth of his organization and for making a generous gesture to that alderman and civil servant.

(re)formulation of professional and functional responsibilities, by short decision making procedures and a small management team at the top, and by re-defining the relations with the municipalities and the role of the board. Besides that he opted for formal decisions inside and outside on long term organizational policies and preferences. And he looked intensively for a strong binding mission statement.

This statement should bind the old and the new professional groups in the GGD, and should be concrete enough for the board and all political and bureaucratic groups and individuals (stockholders and stakeholders) outside the GGD to support the GGD with the desired money and legitimacy.

The CEO had considerable success in handling the conflicting demands of politics and action. To gain legitimacy and other resources, he succeeded in satisfying inconsistent (environmental and internal) norms and producing co-ordinated organizational action simultaneously.

Firstly he started and completed a re-organisation of the GGD in the direction of a modern, rational and action-oriented organization. He reformed the bureaucratic functional organization into a product organization with four departments with different tasks and activities, and a staff to support the CEO and those departments and to improve innovative activities.

The next step was a change of the management structure. Having previously been a broad discussion platform for all sections and disciplines in the organization, the management team became a small decision making group for structural (tactical) and operational matters. Each head of department became responsible for his or her department. This re-organisation resulted in a concentration of professional productive action in four units, and most political type discussions on the new public health ideology and the implementation of these vision in the form of future regular activities in one other unit. The new management team acted as the decision making link for the adaptation of talk into action. So this can be considered as a successful internal separation of politics and action by separation of units.

The CEO did the same with the external separation of politics and action. First he started a planning process for the overall organization and for specific activities. The board took a role in leading and controlling the re-organisation plan and not in discussing national health policies. This meant that a separation of environment for politics and action took place. The municipalities got the politics, the board the (organizational) got the action. From now on different responsibilities and different influences were separated in different environments.

At the same time he started bilateral talks with every municipality separately, supported by members of the management team and the supporting staff. In these talks the representatives of the GGD and a municipality spoke about specific tasks and activities of the GGD, about special problems, interests and wishes of that municipality, but never about central or district health policies or on community prevention ideology in general. All municipalities were very pleased to receive so much attention and they requested bilateral talks on a regular basis instead of negotiations in the district council. This confirmed the role of the board company action-oriented and not as a political platform of municipal representatives. The district council, which was meant to be the political platform of the municipalities, was distanced.

The CEO wrote the overall mission statement himself. To link old, new, external and internal views on topics and options in public health, he formulated a mission statement on the fight against common diseases. This formulation was shown and canvassed to all groups, inside and outside the organization. For politicians it covered different political meanings towards public health sufficiently. It reconciled party political and intra municipal visions and conflicts. For them it functioned also as a kind of decision, directly leading to co-ordinated action (as they thought) by the GGD.

For the different groups of professionals inside the GGD this mission statement reflected enough of their own vision on public health and community prevention to agree on the further plans of their managers for their own departments and units. "It could have been worse", they said.

CONCLUSION

This case description showed us how a CEO of a GGD handled the conflicting demands of politics and action. He was utilizing three or four techniques of separating politics from action at the same time and in a mixture: in different environments, in different organizational units, and by subject matter. In other words, this case showed us how the management of one organization succeeded in satisfying inconsistent (environmental and internal) norms and producing co-ordinated organizational action simultaneously to gain legitimacy and other resources.

In our opinion, Brunssons ideas of incorporating different organizational structures, processes and ideologies for internal and external use (Brunsson 1989), are a promising way to describe and analyse the ways organizations try to achieve organizational legitimacy (and other resources) in a world where organizations are exposed to an increasing number of inconsistent and conflicting norms and demands.

REFERENCES

Berman, P and McLaughlin M.W. (1976), 'Implementation of educational innovation' in: *The educational forum'*, 40-3, 347-370.

Brunsson, N. (1989), *The organisation of hypocrisy; talk, decisions and actions in organisations*, John Wiley Sons, Chichester.

Crown, J. (1990), 'The renaissance of public health', in: De Leeuw, E. (Ed), *Research for healthy cities*, Conference proceedings, the Hague, also available as supplement to *Tijschrift voor Sociale Gezondheidzorg*, vol 86, nr. 11/90.

De Leeuw, E. (1989), *Health policy, an exploratory inquiry into the development of policy for the new public health in the Netherlands*, De Tribune, Maastricht.

De Leeuw, E. (ed.) (1990), *Research for healthy cities,* Conference proceedings, the Hague, also available as supplement to *Tijdschrift voor Sociale Gezondheidszorg,* vol 86, nr. 11/90.

De Leeuw, E. (ed.) (1991), *Gezonde steden; lokale gezondheidsbevordering in theorie, politiek en praktijk,* Van Gorcum, Assen/Maastricht.

De Swaan, A. (1989), *Zorg en de staat,* Bert Bakker, Amsterdam.

Einstadt, S.N. (1968), 'Social institutions', in: *International Encyclopaedia of the Social Sciences,* vol 14, 1968.

Goold, M. and Quinn, J.J. (1990), 'The paradox of strategic controls', in: *Strategic Management Journal,* Vol. 11, 1990, 43-57.

Harrison, M.A. (1987), *Diagnostic organizations; methods, models and processes,* Sage Publ., Newbury Park.

Hofstede, G. (1981), Management control of public and not-for-public activities', in: *Accounting, Organization and Society,* Vol 6, no. 3, 1981, 193-211.

Kaasjager, D.C. (ed.) (1988), *Healthy cities; dageraad van een nieuwe volksgezondheid,* DOP, Den Haag.

Lincoln, Y.S. (ed.) (1985). *Organizational theory and inquiry; the paradigm revolution,* Sage Publ., Newbury Park.

Meijer, A.W.M. (1991), 'Plaats en functies van de Nederlandse GGD-en', in: E. De Leeuw (red): *Gezonde Steden, lokale gezondheidsbevordering in theorie, politiek en praktijk,* Van Gorcum, Assen/Maastricht, 109-132.

Meijer, A.W.M. (1993a), *Ontwikkeling van beleid en organisatie van gezondheidsdiensten; een organisatie-sociologische benadering.* Intern onderzoeksrapport, Maastricht.

Meijer, A.W.M. (1993b), *Ontwikkeling van beleid en organisatie van gezondheidsdiensten; case studies.* Intern onderzoeksrapport, Maastricht.

Meyer, J.W. and Rowan, B. (1977), 'Institutionalized Organizations; formal structure as myth and ceremony', in: *American Journal of Sociology,* Vol. 83, 1977, nr. 2, p. 340-363.

Meyer, J.W. and Scott, W.R. (Ed). (1983), *Organizational environments ritual and rationality,* Sage Publ., Newbury Park.

Peper, B. (1992). *Vorming van welzijnsbeleid, evolutie en evaluatie van het opbouwwerk,* Boom, Meppel.

Perrow, Ch. (1986), *Complex organizations; a critical essay,* Random House, New York.

Pfeffer, J. (1981), *Power in organizations,* Ballinger Publ. Comp., Cambridge Mass.

Pfeffer, J. (1992), *Managing with power; politics and influence in organizations,* Harvard Business and School Press, Boston.

Reed, M.I. (1992), *The sociology of organizations; themes, perspectives and prospects,* Harvester/Wheatsheaf, Hemel Hempstead.

Scott, W.R. (1987), 'The adolescence of institutional theory', in: *Administrative Science Quarterly,* Vol 32., 493-511.

Scott, W.R. (1992), *Organizations; rational, natural and open systems,* Prentice Hall, Englewood Cliffs NJ.

Thompson, J.D. (1967), *Organizations in action,* Mc Graw-Hill, New York.

Timmers, B.P. (1991), *De GGD: Geen gemene deler?,* Doctoraalscriptie Rijksuniversiteit Limburg, Maastricht.

Van de Water, H.P.A. (1989), *Bouwen aan basisgezondheidzorg; over wetenschappelijke en organisatorische grondslagen van collectieve preventie,* NIPG/TNO, Leiden.

Van der West, G. (ed.) (1991), *Vormgeven aan gemeentelijk gezondheidsbeleid. Een kijkje in de keuken,* Van Gorcum, Assen/Maastricht.

Weick, K.E. (1969), *The social psychology of organizing,* Addison-Wesley, Reading Mass.

Zucker, L.G. (ed.) (1988), *Institutional patterns and organizations, culture and environment,* Ballinger Publ. Comp., Cambridge Mass.